Springer Series on

ADULTHOOD and AGING

Series Editors:
Lissy F. Jarvik, M.D., Ph.D., and Bernard D. Starr, Ph.D.

Advisory Board:
Paul D. Baltes, Ph.D., Jack Botwinick, Ph.D., Carl Eisdorfer, M.D., Ph.D., Robert Kastenbaum, Ph.D., Neil G. McCluskey, Ph.D., K. Warner Schaie, Ph.D., and Nathan W. Shock, Ph.D.

Volume 1:
Adult Day Care
Community Work with the Elderly
Philip G. Weiler and Eloise Rathbone-McCuan
with contributors

Volume 2:
Counseling Elders and Their Families
Practical Techniques for Applied Gerontology
John J. Herr and John H. Weakland

Volume 3:
Becoming Old
An Introduction to Social Gerontology
John C. Morgan

Volume 4:
The Projective Assessment of Aging Method (PAAM)
Bernard D. Starr, Marcella Bakur Weiner, and Marilyn Rabetz

Volume 5:
Ethnicity and Aging
Donald E. Gelfand and Alfred J. Kutzik
with 25 contributors

Volume 6:
Gerontology Instruction in Higher Education
David A. Peterson and Christopher R. Bolton

Volume 7:
Nontraditional Therapy and Counseling with the Aging
S. Stansfeld Sargent
with 18 contributors

S. Stansfeld Sargent was awarded his Ph.D. in psychology at Columbia University, where he taught for fifteen years. He later served as a clinical psychologist at the Phoenix VA Hospital, and in the Ventura County (California) Mental Health Department, from which he retired in 1976. He was a founder and vice-chairman of the Ventura County Council on Aging and is now psychological consultant to the Santa Monica Senior Multiservice Center and the Olive Stone Day Activity Center. Dr. Sargent is coauthor of *Basic Teachings of the Great Psychologists* and of a textbook in social psychology and has contributed to many professional journals. He is a former president of the Society for Psychological Study of Social Issues, and of the Association for Humanistic Psychology. He is a diplomate in clinical psychology of the American Board of Professional Psychology, and conducts a small private practice.

NONTRADITIONAL THERAPY AND COUNSELING WITH THE AGING

S. Stansfeld Sargent,
Editor

with contributors

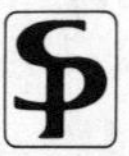

SPRINGER PUBLISHING COMPANY
New York

Springer Publishing Company, Inc.
200 Park Avenue South
New York, New York 10003

80 81 82 83 84 / 10 9 8 7 6 5 4 3 2 1

Library of Congress Cataloging in Publication Data

Main entry under title:

Nontraditional therapy and counseling with the aging.

(Springer series on adulthood and aging; 7)
Bibliography: p.
Includes index.
1. Social work with the aged—United States—Addresses, essays, lectures. 2. Counseling—United States—Addresses, essays, lectures. 3. Psychotherapy—United States—Addresses, essays, lectures.
I. Sargent, Stephen Stansfeld, 1906- II. Series.
[DNLM: 1. Counseling—In old age. 2. Psychology—In old age. 3. Psychotherapy—In old age. WT150 N814]
HV1461.N66 362.6'6 80-11303
ISBN 0-8261-2800-9
ISBN 0-8261-2801-7 pbk.

Printed in the United States of America

Contents

Preface

The editor of this volume happens not to be a trained gerontologist but a clinical and social psychologist who became interested in older people and their problems while he was working in a VA hospital and a community mental health center. He also became acutely aware of their reticence and their defensiveness—in a word, their resistance—in the area of emotional problems. And he was very frustrated by it!

This led to setting up a discussion session at the 1977 convention of the American Psychological Association in San Francisco; it was called "Motivating the Aging for Counseling and Psychotherapy." Participants were Carol J. Dye, Helen Kitzinger, Jeffrey C. Rosenstein, and Arthur N. Schwartz, with S. Stansfeld Sargent chairing the session. The chairman followed this up with a presentation and discussion at the Western Gerontological Society's 1978 meeting in Tucson, on the topic: "Coping with Senior Resistance to Psychotherapy." Both sessions were attended by people who had also encountered the same kind of resistance, and who described some of their efforts to circumvent it. Tentative plans to publish an article on the subject were superseded by a proposal from Springer Publishing Company to expand the material into a volume for their series on Adulthood and Aging.

All the participants in the APA session have contributed papers to the book, and the editor requested reports from several other persons whose activities and programs are nontraditional in form and therapeutic in effect. He thanks all the contributors for their cooperation and congratulates them for their ingenuity and skill in devising ways of bringing therapeutic help to distressed older persons. He is confident that their reports will be interesting and inspiring to our readers.

—S. Stansfeld Sargent

Contributors

Bernice Bratter, whose M.A. is from Azusa Pacific College, is training coordinator and supervisor of the Peer Counseling for Elderly Persons programs of the Santa Monica Bay Area Health Screening Clinic for the Elderly. She is a marriage and family counselor in private practice and has been working with the aging since 1972. She is a founding member of the Older Persons' Information and Counseling Associates (OPICA), a private, nonprofit organization providing counseling and educational services to older persons.

Russell A. Dunckley earned his Ph.D. in clinical psychology at Southern Illinois University in 1975. After completing a year in internship at Camarillo State Hospital in California, he accepted a position at Texas A & M University where he taught graduate level courses in assessment and psychopathology. Dr. Dunckley has also consulted with a rural outreach program in Texas and has conducted state-funded research in aging. In 1979 he became Director of Mental Health Services for the Brazos Valley region of the Texas Department of Mental Health and Mental Retardation.

Carol J. Dye received her Ph.D. in psychology from Washington University. She is now with the Geriatric Research, Education and Clinical Center at the VA Medical Center in St. Louis, and is a research associate in the Aging and Human Development program of the Department of Psychology at Washington University. She has specialized in problems of the elderly in her clinical work, consulting, teaching and research, and has taught courses on aging at most of the universities and colleges in the St. Louis area. Her research reported in this volume resulted from a grant from the National Institute on Aging.

Helena C. Hult has her B.A. degree from Immaculate Heart College in Los Angeles. She retired in 1978 as director of the Senior Service

Center of Santa Monica, and is now president of the consulting firm of Arechaederra-Hult Associates. Previously she was director of the Retired Senior Volunteer Program and of the Volunteer Services at the Santa Monica Hospital Medical Center. She has also been a news reporter and columnist, a secretary and office manager, in addition to raising two children. She was a founding member of the Southern California Society of Directors of Volunteers and of the Santa Monica Westside Volunteer Bureau, and is a board member of the International Association for Volunteer Education.

Helen Kitzinger has her M.A. in clinical psychology from Columbia University. She has been a faculty and board member of Santa Monica Emeritus College since it began in 1974, and is active in volunteer work with the Retired Senior Volunteer Program in the area. Formerly she served as a psychologist at Bellevue Psychiatric Hospital in New York, and at the Sawtelle VA Neuropsychiatric Hospital in Los Angeles. More recently she was a school psychologist for the Santa Monica Unified School District, and a teacher of psychology in the USC Extension Division. She is a diplomate in clinical psychology of the American Board of Professional Psychology.

Robert A. Kooken completed a Bachelor's degree in psychology at Austin College in 1973 and a Master's degree in counseling psychology at Texas A & M University in 1977. He is currently working toward a doctorate in clinical psychology at North Texas State University. Mr. Kooken has worked with the aged through his employment with the Texas Department of Human Resources (program for the aged, blind, and disabled) and through groups he has run for the aged at Texas A & M. He is currently actively involved in research on aging.

Lynn Leonard has a Master of Counseling degree from Arizona State University. She is now Assistant Director, Care/Community Programs of the Foundation for Senior Adult Living in Phoenix, and teaches in the ASU School of Social Work. She was formerly Director of the Retired Senior Volunteer Program in Phoenix, and has been a consultant for city, county, and state personnel departments, and for Sperry Rand Corporation. Ms. Leonard has published articles and presented papers in the areas of counseling and adult day care, and is currently President of the Arizona Association of Adult Day Care Centers.

Candida J. Lutes earned her Ph.D. in developmental psychology at Southern Illinois University in 1976. After teaching for one year at the University of California at Santa Barbara, she has been giving courses in human development and aging at Texas A & M University. Dr. Lutes has also conducted research in aging funded by the Texas Governor's Committee on Aging and the Texas Department of Human Resources, and supervises students working with the aged in nursing homes and retirement communities.

Genevieve R. Meyer was awarded her Ph.D. in psychology by UCLA. She is Associate Professor of Counselor Education at California State University, Los Angeles, where she teaches in the Rehabilitation Counselor Education Program. She gives practicum and testing courses and has developed a class in pre-retirement counseling. She has conducted several workshops and conference presentations on retirement and gerontological counseling, and originated the New Directions Workshop for seniors given under the auspices of the Santa Monica Recreation and Parks Department.

Richard A. Reinhart took his Ph.D. at Western Reserve University. He is Chief Psychologist and leader of the Community Services Team of the Ventura County Mental Health Department. He was previously Supervising Psychologist at the Tompkins County Mental Health Clinic in Ithaca, New York. He has also done public relations and newspaper work, and has contributed to several professional journals. Dr. Reinhart is a diplomate in clinical psychology of the American Board of Professional Psychology, and conducts a part-time private practice.

Cherryl C. Richards was awarded her Ph.D. by Washington University in 1968 in clinical gerontology; she is now a research associate in gerontological psychology with the Department of Psychology at Washington. Previously she was a clinical psychologist with the VA Hospital, Jefferson Barracks, St. Louis, during which time she worked with the aged group of the Nursing Home Care Unit. In 1977 she joined Dr. Dye to work on the research project investigating ways of easing the transition of older people into nursing homes.

Jeffrey C. Rosenstein is Assistant Professor of psychology and coordinator of the Mental Health Specialist Program at California Lutheran College. He was previously a research associate in the Department of Psychiatry, UCLA Medical School–Neuropsychiatric Institute, and associate director of the Behavior Analysis and Modification in Community Mental Health Centers Project. He is a doctoral candidate in social psychology at the Claremont Graduate School.

Arthur N. Schwartz was granted the Ph.D. by Washington University in St. Louis. Since 1970 he has been very much involved with the Andrus Gerontology Center of the University of Southern California, as Adjunct Professor of Psychology and as director of the Adult Counseling Training Program. He has also served in training and consultant activities on aging with many community agencies, and conducts a private clinical practice. Dr. Schwartz has published widely in the field of aging, two of his most recent books being *Survival Handbook for Children of Aging Parents* and *Introduction to Gerontology* (co-author).

Edwin W. Swenson was awarded his Ph.D. in clinical psychology at the University of Utah. He is Professor of Psychology at California Lutheran College, and Assistant Research Psychologist, UCLA Medical School–Neuropsychiatric Institute. Previously, he was Director of the UCLA Family Learning Center. He was also Assistant Research Psychologist of the UCLA Behavior Analysis and Modification Project.

Estelle Tuvman received her M.P.H. degree from California State University at Northridge. She is presently the Administrative Director of the Santa Monica Bay Area Health Screening Clinic for the Elderly, Inc., and wrote the grant proposal for Peer Counseling for the Elderly (PEP). She is a former consultant to the Los Angeles Unified School District, Special Education Division.

John M. Vayhinger has a B. D. from Drew Theological Seminary, and a Ph.D. in psychology from Columbia University. He is Professor of Psychology and Pastoral Care and department chairman at the Anderson (Indiana) School of Theology. He has served as pastor of several Methodist churches, and has taught pastoral psychology and counseling at Northwestern University and the University of Denver. He has done psychological research on the theological student, and is director of a workshop in mental health for the clergy, which is supported by grants from the National Institute for Mental Health. Dr. Vayhinger is a diplomate in clinical psychology of the American Board of Professional Psychology, and conducts a part-time private practice.

Eugenie G. Wheeler received her M.S.W. at the New York School of Social Work. Since 1970 she has been a Senior Psychiatric Social Worker with the Ventura County Department of Mental Health. Previously she was Staff Development Supervisor of the Ventura County Department of Social Welfare, and a curriculum coordinator for the U.C. Santa Barbara Extension Certificate Program in the Social Services. She cooperated in developing a new format for group marriage counseling and has contributed to symposia and publications. She conducts a private practice and has led many groups on assertiveness training and anxiety management for women and for older people.

Judith N. Wooten completed a Bachelor's degree at Texas A & M University in 1973, and a Master's degree in counseling psychology at Texas A & M in 1975. She is currently completing a doctoral degree in counseling at Texas A & M. Ms. Wooten's work in aging includes groups, individual and couple therapy with aged clients, consultation with community agencies that provide services to elders, and research on sexuality and aging.

Introduction: Why Nontraditional Therapy and Counseling with the Aging?

S. Stansfeld Sargent

Someone may ask "But why therapy or counseling for the aging at all? What's the point?"

It's true that there are more than 30 million persons over 60 in the United States, and most of them are active and functioning well. But some, as in any other group in our population, have distressing emotional problems that they seem unable to solve by themselves—problems like depression, intense fears, anxiety, persistent anger, frustration, unrelieved loneliness. And others have occasional problems which are too much for them, especially grief and depression caused by the death of a loved one.

"All right then, why don't they get help from a psychologist or a psychiatrist or go to a mental health clinic like anybody else?"

A good question. They should, because there are many professional and other trained people who could probably aid them. But the plain fact is *most older people don't and won't ask for help with their emotional problems. They resist.* They not only won't ask, but many of them won't accept assistance if and when it is offered.

That's where the nontraditional approaches come in. "Nontraditional" psychotherapy or counseling is a term used to cover many programs and approaches which are therapeutic and which older people can accept.*

Let's go back a little, and be more specific.

In our country people usually enter retirement with mixed feelings. Many are glad to leave behind the routine of their work and look forward to recreation, relaxation, travel, a chance to indulge in their hobbies, and the like. Most are in good health and expect to live many years. They know they will have to get along on a smaller income but feel they can manage all right. Surveys show that the recently retired are reasonably happy and well satisfied with life.

But retirees soon become conscious of problems that are faced by older people in our society. For example:

- Too often they are regarded as being "on the shelf," "put out to pasture," or fifth wheels no longer of much significance.
- They no longer work, and they become aware that society disapproves of anyone who is not productive; in fact, deep down, they too disapprove!
- The awful combination of diminished income and relentless inflation slowly gets through to them, and they begin to wonder if they will be able to make it.

Added to these are problems faced by older people everywhere, notably:

- They realize they have entered the last stage of life and they come to think of the future in a different way, in terms of "How much time do I have left?"
- They encounter physical limitations and restrictions, with increasing incidence of chronic illness and disability.
- They experience devastating losses, through death or serious illness, of spouses, close relatives and friends, colleagues and associates.

Older people probably have more psychological problems than any other age group, except possibly adolescents, though it is difficult to prove this statement conclusively. However, there is much relevant evidence.

In 1974, 25 percent of the patients in state and county mental hospitals were persons over 65, as compared with their actual 10 percent of the U.S. population (Butler and Lewis, 1977). Another study found that those over 65 account for about one-quarter of new

*The writer is indebted to Dr. Arthur Schwartz for suggesting the use of "nontraditional" in this connection.

admissions to state mental hospitals (Shanas and Maddox, 1976); some other researchers have arrived at higher percentages.

The American Psychological Association has estimated that 15 percent of the older population need mental health services. Others consider this too conservative a figure. Butler and Lewis would place it much higher. They would include many persons with chronic physical illness because of associated emotional reactions. They would also add the millions of aged who live at or below the poverty level "in conditions that are known to contribute to emotional breakdown or decline" (Butler and Lewis, 1977, p. 52).

Another estimate states that among those over 65 living in the community, about 5 percent are severely impaired in psychological functioning, and a further 20 percent moderately impaired (Shanas and Maddox, 1976). However, largely due to the shift of older people from hospitals to nursing homes, they are less likely to have help now than formerly, concludes one investigator. "Rather than helping older persons, the great mental health revolution has only led to their dropping out of the psychiatric system. Certainly the new programs have not helped the aged" (Kahn, 1975, p. 25).

And finally, in the United States 25 percent of the suicides are committed by persons over 65, particularly by white males, whose figure is far above any other group (Butler, 1976).

Thus, the evidence seems overwhelming that a great many older people are emotionally upset and could benefit from some kind of therapeutic help. But what do we find? Several studies of the clientele of mental health clinics and of private practitioners have shown that only a very small percentage (between 1 and 5 percent) are persons over 60 years of age (e.g., Buckley, 1977; Kahn, 1975). This means that most of the older people with problems simply are not coming for help, despite the large number who have been discharged from state and county hospitals and returned to their home communities, usually with the understanding that they will continue to receive treatment on an outpatient basis. What has gone wrong?

Many gerontologists feel that the community mental health centers and clinicians generally have fallen down on the job and are not interested in trying to help older people. Indeed it has been said that many professionals share the myths and misunderstandings of what Dr. Robert Butler calls "ageism" (Butler and Lewis, 1977, pp. 141–142). This refers to prejudice and discrimination on the part of the middle-aged and the young against the old, reflecting a deep-seated distaste and even revulsion against growing old and becoming diseased or disabled.

Undoubtedly one can find among professional therapists and counselors, as among the population at large, many examples of stereotypes about the elderly: "they're rigid"; "they won't change"; or even "I'm busy and I haven't time for 'old crocks.'" However, there are signs that the professionals are becoming more aware of the problems of the aging and are willing to work with them (see Dye, 1978). Probably a typical attitude is, "I'd be glad to try to help these older folks, if they'd only come in!"

Reasons for the Resistance

"If they'd only come in." This is the crux of the problem, a sign of the attitude noted by practically everyone who works with older people, and by a few researchers as well—a tremendous resistance to psychotherapy and considerable resistance to counseling or any form of behavior change. This is particularly evident if the therapist suggested is a psychiatrist or a clinical psychologist, or a staff member of a mental health center. It is difficult to know just why this resistance occurs, but several plausible reasons have been advanced by people in the field.

One of the most frequent explanations is that the aging are more independent or "inner-directed" than others, which makes them ashamed to ask for help. Buckley thinks that our older people, especially those born before or soon after 1900, need to see themselves as strong and self-sufficient, as they were in their younger days. So they deny any need for help and keep their fears and other feelings to themselves. Seeking counseling would be an admission of weakness. They are caught in a cultural lag between their old behavior patterns and the problems of today (Buckley, 1977). Dr. Stephen Soreff, a psychiatrist in Portland, Maine, commented thus on old New England Yankees: "They try to keep it all in, try to be strong, hide their feelings. . . . They feel that to get help for their depression or mental problems is not only wrong, but a symbol of weakness" (report in the *Los Angeles Times,* March 23, 1978). In all fairness, one might comment that this independent spirit, which very likely traces to colonial and pioneer days in American history, may have helped our oldsters to solve problems successfully in their younger years.

Other suggested reasons include:

1. The aging have unfavorable stereotypes of "head doctors" and mental health efforts, possibly originating in childhood impressions of sixty or more years ago about "lunatic asylums" where "insane" people were "committed" by doctors and judges and kept for years, perhaps as long as they lived. These views are often reinforced by gossip and hearsay from family members and friends.

2. Rightly or wrongly, some older people sense a lack of interest in them on the part of clinicians, which increases their resistance to psychiatric or psychological help and at the same time reinforces any negative impressions held by those professionals. An unhappy example, indeed, of a vicious circle!

3. Many older people are unhappy about the rapid changes that have been occurring in our world and end up opposing any kind of change, including changes in their own behavior or personality. Why tackle something questionable and unpleasant, they reason, especially when "I haven't much time left."

4. Some aging persons feel guilty, worthless, and undeserving of help. Dr. Elizabeth Forsberg, a Vermont psychiatrist, described old people this way: "Their insistence at trying to solve their own problems is frequently mixed with a deep feeling that they are no longer useful to society. And this combination all too often leads them to suicide" (*Los Angeles Times,* March 23, 1978).

5. They don't know to whom to turn for help, or they don't know how much it might cost and whether it would be covered by Medicare or other insurance they might have.

6. Some are tied down by home cares or illness, are tired or unable to move about easily, or lack transportation.

Of course, as we have already indicated, a few seniors *do* have professional psychotherapy or counseling, and their record for being helped is favorable (see Blau and Berezin, 1975; Butler and Lewis, 1977, Chap. 12). Once they are motivated and have overcome their resistance, they can very probably benefit as much as younger people.

Enter the Nontraditional Therapist

There is accumulating evidence that older people are often aided therapeutically by persons untrained as counselors or therapists, or by professionals using newer kinds of approaches. Perhaps it is a close friend or relative who listens sympathetically, reassures, suggests and encourages activities, remains in contact, and helps pull the new widow out of her depression. Or again, a nurse or social worker may turn her association with the senior into therapeutic directions without evoking resistance and may help the individual to gain insight, a new resolve, a wish to change, a gradual return to social life in the community.

As we shall see, the peer counseling program for seniors is carried on by volunteers who are seniors themselves and who, after some training, are able to help many kinds of distressed older persons in their community. They are accepted because they are perceived as being the same kind of people as the counselees. Other older volunteers, such as those with the Retired Senior Volunteer Program (RSVP), are supplied to community agencies to provide much-needed services of many sorts. These volunteers not only give valuable community service, but they benefit emotionally from the experience of aiding others—as the originators of the RSVP foresaw.

A discussion group on seniors' problems may or may not go in a direction which could be called therapeutic. Sometimes it becomes a sounding board for a few very articulate individuals or serves to focus advocacy or protest. Or it might function at an informative or intellectual level, like a class, or turn its efforts toward finding solutions for one or more substantive problems. On the other hand, a discussion group or social club, with guidance from the leader, may become in effect a therapy group, with thc members expressing pent-up feelings, reaching out to help each other, communicating, empathizing, and working to formulate plans for better living.

The editor is psychological consultant for a multiservice center for seniors. He discovered long ago that identifying himself as a clinical psychologist could be very threatening to some of the people. However, if he were introduced as a "research psychologist who is interested in the life stories of older people," a potential negative reaction could turn into a positive one. And within half an hour a life story interview could become a genuinely therapeutic session.

These are but a few examples of nontraditional psychotherapy or counseling, which tends to be indirect and informal, growing out of natural or conventional social relationships. Much detailed description and many cases will be given in the chapters of this book. The necessary condition for beneficial change, of course, is basically *rapport*—an empathic and trusting relationship between two individuals or between an individual and the members of a group.

Who Are the Nontraditional Therapists?

Who are some of the people who can best establish this rapport with distraught older persons? It might be the family doctor or the minister, whom many studies have shown to be the persons most often called on by distressed people. Or it might be an old friend and confidant, or a relative who has been trusted and admired over the years. But a lonely and isolated old person may turn to a welfare worker, a visiting nurse, an assigned houseworker, or a friendly volunteer and, if given the least bit of interest and encouragement, may pour out a torrent of pent-up feelings and frustrations, and then feel much better.

But, one may ask, are people like this willing and able to help older persons with their problems? Maybe—and maybe not. The doctor is probably too busy, with a full waiting room and emergencies to handle. Some ministers are indeed attuned to pastoral or personal counseling, while others cleave to their more traditional religious role. Relatives and friends sometimes hesitate to get involved with personal or family matters. Many kinds of workers visit homes or perform personal services; it depends upon their interests, their maturity and experience, and their training, whether or not they wish to essay a therapeutic role.

A social work study was made of "natural helping networks," which can be found in all communities—urban, suburban, and rural. The networks included relatives, friends, and associates, as might be expected. But it turned out that the central figure might be a bartender, beautician, druggist, custodian, or even a gas meter reader! The outstanding traits in the successful helpers were great social interest, empathy, and "freedom from drain," by which the investigators meant without fear of becoming depleted or exhausted (Collins and Pancoast, 1976).

For most helpers, however, training is crucial. Many who work with older people are experienced in listening to and communicating with their clients and want to help them, but they are aware of their lack of training in therapeutic techniques. They wonder if they can get the kind of training which would help them to work more effectively with older persons.

The answer is definitely affirmative.

Many years ago psychologist Margaret Rioch surprised her professional colleagues by showing that a group of mature and interested, but untrained, housewives could become psychotherapists after completing a part-time two-year program of supervised study and practice of psychotherapy. Evaluation revealed that their performance was equal to that of psychiatric residents, graduate students in clinical psychology, and psychoanalytic institute candidates. In fact, they all got jobs in mental health agencies (Rioch et al., 1963).

A later study sponsored by the National Institute of Mental Health reported on no less than 10,000 "paraprofessionals"—meaning persons who work alongside, in cooperation with, professionals. They functioned in individual counseling, various kinds of group therapy, screening, tutoring, and helping people adjust to community life (Sobey, 1970). This does not mean that all paraprofessionals are effective, of course, in providing therapeutic assistance. Training and supervision were found to be "crucial to growth and utilization of inherent skills" (Butler and Lewis, 1977, p. 151).

Many programs have been set up for training volunteers and nonprofessionals to counsel the aging. Probably the best organized are the peer counseling efforts already operating in many communities. One will be described in this book, along with the kind of training received by peer counselors. A well-planned program has been instituted at the Continuum Center of Oakland University in Michigan (Waters and White, 1977). Many other projects are burgeoning, including training for policemen, foremen, bartenders, barbers, beauticians, ex-patients, and others (see Gershon and Biller, 1977).

In a look ahead to the year 2000, Kahn foresees a much more important role for nonprofessionals, "preferably coming from the same background, same neighborhood, and same general age group as the prospective clients." They would be the first line of contact, serving at least in a 'confidant' role and providing liaison to professionals. The latter would provide direct service only to a small number of persons, but serve as *indirect* consultants to "firing line professionals such as police, clergymen, general physicians, and to others such as bank tellers, bus drivers and storekeepers." Most persons, the writer concludes, could be helped without ever becoming officially a "patient" or a "client" (Kahn, 1975).

Why Not Just Call It "Serving" or "Helping"?

About now some readers may be thinking, "Why so much talk about *psychotherapy* and *counseling?* Why imply these old people are abnormal? They just have problems, some of which are of course emotional, for which they sometimes need aid. But why can't we just call it 'serving' or 'helping' or 'assisting'—or even 'befriending'?"

Obviously people are not abnormal because they have an emotional problem for which they need help now and then, and many authorities would not use the term "abnormal" even for the smaller number who have certain kinds of persisting emotional difficulties.

It is often hard to find terms which are satisfactory. "Therapy" means treatment—any kind of remedial or curative treatment. "Psychotherapy" means treatment for emotional or psychological problems. ("Therapy" is often used as a shortened form of "psychotherapy," though there are many other kinds of therapy, such as physical and occupational therapy.) In the United States "counseling" usually means helping people with personal or adjustment problems, and it becomes very difficult to draw a line between counseling and psychotherapy.

Some might prefer to describe the essential process as "change," since change in behavior or personality is implied in both psychotherapy and counseling. But the term "change" covers too much ground. Similarly, words like "helping" or "assisting" are descriptive, but very broad. "Befriending" is used a great deal in England, connoting a sympathetic, listening, and helping attitude on the part of volunteers. It is the central theme of the suicide prevention work of the Samaritans (see Varah, 1965), but the term has not caught on widely in the U.S.

Another slight semantic problem is that neither "psychotherapy" nor "counseling," strictly speaking, includes the *prevention* of mental illness, which is of great concern to many aging persons. Nor do the two words cover the "self-actualization" of the humanistic psychologist, who use this term for all persons who are seeking to realize their full growth or potential, whether or not they are plagued by emotional problems.

However, all the terms we have mentioned are oriented toward aiding the person to cope, to avoid emotional stress, to improve, to grow, to become fulfilled. Insofar as the contact is made indirectly and informally, in innovative and nonthreatening fashion, especially by persons other than professionals, we lump it under the head of "nontraditional therapy" (or "nontraditional counseling"). These terms may well change and be superseded by others, but for the present we find them useful to cover several new approaches and programs for aiding distressed older people.

Now That Term "Therapeutic"

We still need to define more precisely that we mean by the concept "therapeutic." Actually, any activity or human contact which pleases older people, channels their energies, increases their skills, gets them outdoors, enables them to make new friends, and exposes them to new experiences might be considered "therapeutic." But this is too broad; it includes almost the whole range of senior activities—educational, recreational, social, and physical. If our concept is not more definite than this, we shall get nowhere.

To be quite specific, let us say that a contact or experience has been therapeutic if it results in certain kinds of beneficial changes in the person. Probably the most obvious of these changes is a decrease in upsetting symptoms and complaints, such as depression, anxiety, anger, loneliness, or whatever distressed the person previously. But there are many other evidences of therapeutic gain; for example:

- Improvement in appearance, manner, dress, eating or sleeping habits, interest in things, and more *joie de vivre* in general;
- Talking out feelings, frustrations, and problems and working toward solving them;
- Increased attention to other persons, showing empathy, moving away from self-centeredness;
- Interest in helping others, and taking steps to do something about it;
- Signs of insight and perspective; more balance and tolerant views of self, others, and the community;
- Signs of increasing autonomy, independence, self-direction, assertiveness, and improved self-image;
- Any creative activity, whether in arts, crafts, ideas, plans for neighborhood or community improvement, or other areas;
- Growing awareness of the environment and of changes occurring in the world; moves toward participation and involvement in wider contexts.

Overview of the Book

Because the problems are so pressing, many workers with older people have been devising programs of a nontraditional sort to help them cope with their anxiety, frustration, depression, anger, loneliness, boredom, and assorted psychosomatic problems. Literally hundreds of attempts have been made, and are being made, to provide therapeutic help for our older citizens who are upset and unhappy. Sometimes these efforts have been made by professionals who have modified and disguised the traditional approaches in order to circumvent the typical senior resistance. Sometimes the approach has been made by people with little or no professional training who have great empathy and who are close to the lives and problems of older people.

But, so far as the editor is aware, no systematic attempt has been made to collect, analyze, and interpret these varied therapeutic efforts. This is the task which is begun in this volume, with several descriptive reports and illustrative cases straight from "where the action is" in cities, towns, and rural areas of our country.

Because of our hope that the book will be of practical value to those working with the aging, the contributors are describing their orientation, programs, and activities in some detail. Evidence of therapeutic change is found in both objective and subjective data, a good deal of it in the form of cases cited. Examples of failure or of very modest success are sometimes given, especially where there is some understanding of the causes. Obviously no effort will be therapeutic for everyone; some authorities would say that noticeable improvement in 5 or 10 percent of a sizable group of people is very good. We might go further and say that if a program is clearly beneficial for even *one* participant, it has the potential to be so for others. This should encourage workers with the aging who are planning to set up new programs or to make existing ones more appealing and effective.

The first six of the nontraditional programs described here represent new approaches on the part of professionals, generally within the framework of existing senior service facilities in the community. The next three chapters deal with volunteers, their supervision, and their training. Three other reports illustrate the application of particular psychological viewpoints—the humanistic, the behavioral, and the pastoral—in helping seniors deal with their emotional problems.

Since our emphasis is upon the active, noninstitutionalized older person, we have not described therapeutic programs within the hospital setting, such as occupational therapy, physical therapy, or music and art therapy. These therapies are beginning to spread into the day care and day activity programs of senior centers, and reports of their therapeutic value in the wider community setting should be forthcoming in the near future.

In a word, our book is not about the "traditional" psychotherapy and counseling which is being performed, by professionals, for a disconcertingly small percentage of older people. Instead, we provide a dozen reports from workers directly involved in providing "nontraditional" therapeutic services, which are more acceptable to that sizable minority of our older population who have psychological problems or who are striving for change, growth, and fulfillment in their lives.

Part I

Nontraditional Therapy in the Setting of Senior Services

1

Assertive Training Groups for the Aging

Eugenie G. Wheeler

What Is Assertive Training?

"There are no quick rewards for the depressed person. It is a matter of making a channel and then guiding one's boat through it, day by day" (Sarton, 1968). Assertive training is a unique approach to helping older people carve out a channel or pathway to behavior change and to change in their experience of being older.

Assertiveness, as it is used in this context, is the happy medium between passivity and aggressiveness. To be passive is to allow your rights to be violated, or to violate your own rights, or perhaps not even to recognize that you have personal rights. To be aggressive is to violate the rights of others. To be assertive is to communicate directly with no put-downs of yourself or others. Assertive training is based on a recognition of human rights—our own and those of others. Skills in assertive communication are uniquely effective for the elderly in dealing with the put-downs they are subjected to.

Assertive training is a relatively new approach to helping people improve their communication skills. It focuses on building mutually respectful social interactions through modeling, role-playing, and positive feedback or reinforcement. It is based on the theory that passivity or aggressiveness in social relations leads to anxiety, depression, and low self-esteem, while one is more able to fulfill one's own needs when one takes an assertive stance. Clients are taught to express their feelings in direct, honest ways but without accusations or hostility. Central to the method is involving the participants in role-playing scenes in which the participants rehearse incidents in relationships they wish to improve. Sometimes a hierarchy of scenes is developed involving ascending levels of emotional threat and learning difficulty. Only when clients satisfactorily carry out a situation in "real life" do they move to the next step up in the hierarchy.

Esquire, in its humorous advice on how to grow old, advises, "Rage, don't whine." Raging is aggressive, whining is passive. There is a whole range of possible behaviors in between, and clients can be helped to enhance their repertoires of behaviors and to be aware of their choices through assertive training groups with modeling and behavior rehearsal.

Why Assertive Training for the Aging?

In our culture today the elderly are often relegated to the sidelines, but it is also true that at times elderly persons allow themselves to be too easily pushed aside. They may be conniving a little in their own relegation through their passivity (Tournier, 1972). Others among the elderly hold resentments inside too long (as do all ages), letting the hurts and indignities fester until they can no longer be held in. Then it all comes out inappropriately, or aggressively, and elderly persons are not likely to get what they want, or to feel good about it.

Assertive training can provide ways for aging individuals to express their feelings directly as they come up. This is a way to prevent depression because when put-downs or slights are countered, they are not internalized and do not eat away at the self-image.

Arthur Schwartz (1977) points out that if older persons are treated persistently in a patronizing manner, as if they were not-too-bright children, if options are removed by others who take complete control, if older people are continually demeaned and belittled and treated coldly and with indifference (whether that happens quite openly or very subtly), you can bet that some senile-like behavior is likely to occur. Some old people will fight back, but others will lapse into senile/passive behavior. In other words, if middle-agers treat their elderly parents and others as if they were entering a second childhood, you will most likely see a self-fulfilling prophecy. Aggressiveness teaches passivity.

Butler and Lewis (1977) describe the sense of helplessness that occurs when one is old and ill or incapacitated. There is often inadequate opportunity to be assertive in a way that alleviates this feeling. A bedridden person, for example, may finally resort to purposely urinating in bed to vent angry feelings.

Although assertive training can be effective with a wide variety of target groups, there are several reasons why this approach has special appeal and relevance to older people:

- It is skills training.
- It is practical.
- It is best done in groups with informality and humor.

Assertive training as skills training. Assertiveness is perceived as a skill rather than as a personality attribute. To have as a goal the learning of a new skill is far less threatening than trying to achieve a change in one's basic personality. Assertive training does not carry with it the implication that the participant is "sick" or maladjusted. It is rather that we have often learned to be passive or aggressive in certain situations where it is inappropriate. The assertive training group can help us unlearn these behaviors and learn instead better ways of interacting and communicating.

Assertive training is practical. With assertive training no one is going to be "fooling around" with the aging person's so-called unconscious. This approach sounds like commonsense to older people, who are not used to joining therapy groups or articulating their feelings. Assertive training deals in practical ways with day-to-day situations that are of concern in the present and the immediate future.

Assertive training as fun. Most older people like the informality; they can "play act" in easy role-playing situations, and there is plenty of room for humor. Assertive training groups are geared to education, support, socialization, and skills training. They are non-threatening, are only mildly confrontative, do not attack defenses, and are conducive to feelings of pride, accomplishment, and growth.

Often seniors will come to an assertive training group when they will not come to one labeled a "therapy" group. If they resist an assertive training group because they confuse the terms *assertive* and *aggressive,* titles such as "personal effectiveness" or "communication training" are perfectly acceptable. The point is that assertive training, whatever it is called, can help older people accept aging without accepting "ageism," and, counter put-downs instead of integrating them into their self-image. It can help them rid themselves of their own inner restrictive assumptions about aging. We are all, after all, products of our culture, and if we are honest with ourselves, we will recognize that we are still subject to some of the cultural myths about aging—that newness, speed, and youthfulness are somehow better. After participating in an assertive training group, a person feels less vulnerable to such myths whether they are on the inside or the outside. When other group members share and model scenes illustrating that there is more than one effective way to express feelings, and that there is a wide range of choices on the behavioral continuum from passive to aggressive, the learning of these options diminishes the participants' feelings of helplessness and anxiety and increases their confidence and effectiveness.

A "Self-Esteem Group"

Background

The Oxnard Outpatient Clinic of the Ventura County Health Services Agencies was having the same experience as other clinics throughout the country in terms of the numbers of elderly people applying for help. Most reports indicate that people over 65 make up 19 percent of all admissions to state and county mental hospitals, but only 2 percent of all patients admitted to psychiatric outpatient clinics. Several attempts had been made to reach distressed older people. Some were successful and some were not.

In the early 1970s, two members of the outpatient staff planned for a group of seniors to meet away from the clinic to avoid the stigma, with some transportation help from the Welfare Department. It was felt that by holding the therapy sessions in a neutral setting (a bank was selected) and by having the participants brought to the sessions, some of the major problems would be overcome. The group was entitled "The Group for Actualizing Senior Potential" (acronym: The GASP Group) and was to be co-led by a psychologist and a social worker. It was not considered to be a successful venture, but much was learned from the experience that is now being put to use. The learning may be summarized as:

1. Many of the elderly do, in fact, resist going to a Mental Health Clinic for help because of the stigma, and inner restrictive assumptions such as that it means one is "crazy."

2. Lack of transportation is, indeed, a factor in the underutilization of the resources of the clinic.

3. Lack of knowledge of the resources is a third element that needs to be overcome.

4. Adequate screening for referral to a group is essential and should include consideration of:

- the "sore thumb" principle. This means there should not be any member so different from the rest that he or she stands out like a sore thumb; for example, if all are college educated, one person with only a third grade education might feel uncomfortable.
- the ability to listen and to hear as well as to talk. These abilities should be verified before acceptance into a group.
- an attention span that allows for a level of communication. This should be decided upon in advance.
- the preparation that should be given prior to the beginning of the group. For example, ground rules regarding confidentiality, acceptable feedback, and attendance.

A more successful program was an agency-based Senior Group co-led by two social workers that has become an ongoing support group of six to eight participants. The leaders provide insight therapy, assertive training, self-esteem-raising interventions, and much crisis-intervention-type problem-solving. The members themselves have renamed this group the "Talk Show" and are finding it to be a significant part of their lives. The learning acquired from this experience was applied to the Assertive Training Group which was later established. This learning can be summarized as follows:

1. Co-leadership has many advantages for such a group in setting an "up" tone and providing balance, coverage, training, and richer feedback.

2. Seniors can make effective use of a wide variety of modalities in group therapy, including assertive training.

3. There must be allowance for a great deal of mutual support-giving and problem-solving to get maximum participation and benefit.

An "over 50s" group for women aged 50 and above has also been successful and has further substantiated how effective group therapy can be with groups of older people.

But the question remained of how to reach more of them, the ones with transportation difficulties and the ones with the many kinds of resistance discussed in the introduction to this book; the ones that just don't come. It was felt that an outreach program at a site where the Senior Nutrition Program was serving lunches to seniors would have many advantages as a place to start, the chief one being that the seniors were already *there.*

The idea for a Counseling Information program at a Senior Nutrition meal site emerged out of discussions among social workers and Senior Nutrition Program staff, and at the meetings of the Community Services Committee on Services to the Aged. The possibility of a pilot project was discussed with all of the staff that would be involved, and a meal site was selected based on requests from Senior Nutrition staff, size of the group served, and estimates regarding the potential success of the program. An announcement was made at the site that counseling would be available on Wednesdays, 11:00–1:00, in four half-hour sessions. The site manager agreed to keep an appointment schedule. The plan was to screen clients for referral to an Assertive Training Group or to the outpatient clinic or to other appropriate community resources, depending on the need. In the meantime, the social worker went to the site every Wednesday to get to know the potential clients informally. Every Wednesday the social worker made an announcement that the service was available, and every time she did the announcement was met with enthusiastic applause. However, the only ones who asked to see her were those who had sat at the same table and talked with her over lunch. Just when there seemed to be a nucleus, some potential group members would "peter out"—that is, move away or fail to attend or become ill.

Getting Started

We wanted to have the group begin before Christmas since the holidays can be an especially difficult time for many of the elderly because of losses in their lives. An adequate nucleus of members failed to develop because so many cases petered out so rapidly, if they moved away from the lunch tables at all. A new approach was started November 2, 1977, and the name was changed. The group leader announced that a "Self-Esteem Group" would be starting on November 30th to meet on Wednesdays from 11:00–12:00. If we had waited for proper screening procedures to take place before taking the plunge it is doubtful that the project would ever have gotten off the ground because many who were interested and in need remained tentative. Some members asked if they could sit in once or twice before deciding whether they would become a part of the group. Others never showed up after promising to do so. The location itself provided a kind of screening because only ambulatory, noninstitutionalized aged who were motivated and able to get to a Senior Meal Program were invited to join. At the same time, the fact that it was located right next to a dining room eliminated the privacy or anonymity that another location might have provided. The setup lent itself to a kind of casualness about attendance that was difficult to combat. It was given as a free "community service," which also may have accounted for the lack of commitment on the part of many.

The group was held from November 30th through the middle of April. Attendance was sporadic in spite of various attempts to get commitments of regular attendance from the participants. Reasons given for absences included family obligations during the holidays, lack of transportation, illness of self and family members, and a feeling on the part of some that their need was not as great as others or sufficient to warrant their coming. The numbers varied from three to fourteen, and this spotty attendance interfered with the continuity and cohesiveness that was needed for full therapeutic benefit.

Some were "fade-outs" who never got to the group. One woman sat down opposite the counselor at lunch saying she was in a real panic about the number of relatives who were arriving for Thanksgiving. She discussed it in low tones so her 87-year-old husband, who was sitting nearby, wouldn't hear. She was understandably anxious not to burden him with her dilemma. She had some good reasons for not wanting to say "no" to her sons. One had gone through a divorce and was bringing his three children. This elderly woman had stayed awake most of the night worrying about her problem and really needed to talk about it. But she did not elect to join the group.

Another woman with a somewhat hysterical manner said she had a problem: She won at bingo, it had been a tie, and both winners agreed to tossing a coin to determine who should get the prize. She had won, the other woman was angry with her, what should she do? The counselor is still not sure how serious the woman was or in what way she, the counselor, was being tested.

Then there was Corinne, 72, who was depressed, but one week later had recovered. She had gone to work for two days. She is a kitchenware demonstrator, and to be called to work had given her an emotional and financial boost. Her husband had refused to allow her to work because of her high blood pressure, but seeing how happy it made her, he had come around to valuing her occasional kitchenware demonstration projects. Her husband, who wandered in at the end of the interview, was referred to the representative from Welfare for help with his application for Supplemental Security Income (SSI). He refused to join the group. Corinne had benefited from the first informal contact at lunch, when she ventilated many of her frustrations at having moved to this area from Minneapolis and at having found it much less advantageous than they had anticipated. Their son and daughter-in-law were not being attentive, housing was unsatisfactory, their new friends did not have the same recreational interests, etc. She had definitely planned to join the group but work intervened.

Another example was Joe, age 77, who, while standing on the food line with the counselor, explained that he had needed the service desperately seventeen months ago when his wife died. He agreed to come to group but two weeks later said he no longer needed help because since the last contact he had become engaged to be married. He rejected offers of premarital counseling or group.

Another woman, over lunch, expressed her rage and anger at having to curtail her activities because of her husband's heart attacks. She implied that she believed he had caused the last one. "He didn't *have* to work in the yard and pick vegetables the day before I was to leave for a trip to see my daughter." Since she had transportation and part-time work and since she appeared to need more intensive help, she was referred to the clinic.

How the Self-Esteem Group Worked

There was a nucleus of four to six members who stayed with it, and one married couple, Bill and Elaine, never missed a session. If a more careful screening job had been achieved, married couples would not have been accepted in the same group. But then we would have lost Bill or Elaine!

The physical setting left something to be desired. It was large and barnlike, with straight, uncomfortable chairs. Often participants were late through no fault of their own as most were dependent on others for rides. Some became restless toward 12:00 because they wanted to be sure of getting their seats early for lunch. In spite of all this, the meetings were exciting, with broad and enthusiastic participation and much personal growth.

The format included an "opener" or warm-up exercise, reports on assignments, some role-playing, new self-assignments, and sometimes a closing exercise. It seemed important to start with less self-revealing activities and work up gradually to more charged material. Openers were for socialization, self-awareness and identity, self-esteem, and goal-setting. Often an opener led right into role-playing. For example, participants might be asked to tell of an incident in which they had been assertive and then a situation in which more assertive skill would be desirable, like "I need to ask my neighbor for a ride but I'm reluctant to." This sort of opening exercise provided opportunities for fruitful behavior rehearsal. An opener that required sentence completion such as, "I would like to learn to . . ." was a natural for self-assignments. These included taking a speed reading course, making an Easter cake, and applying to be a foster grandparent.

Christmas was used for show-and-tell. Group members were invited to bring in samples of the handicrafts they were engaged in, and this served many purposes. It provided opportunities for much genuine positive feedback, it led to New Year's resolutions (goal-setting) regarding next projects, and it also contributed to feelings of achievement and self-worth. Elaine brought drawings done before and after her stroke, Lola brought mirrors framed in sea shells, and there were carpentry items, a quilt, poetry, preserves, and some very fine embroidery.

At one session the group was divided into pairs and after a few minutes of dialogue, the members introduced their partners by repeating three things each one liked about the partner and one thing each member would like to work on for himself or herself. Another opener was a simple awareness exercise which required a list of five words that describe "you." These included: neat, fairly good, patient, on time, artistic, sociable, impatient, overanxious, determined, active, happy, good grandma, sympathetic, good storyteller, too fast for accuracy, Jack-of-all-trades, music lover, nature lover, aggressive, honest, archer, dog lover, knitter, Christian, friendly, etc. One day we all did self-portraits which were revealing in regard to self-concepts.

At subsequent meetings we had the "mastery" or "achievement" exercise where members were asked to recall an incident in their lives that gave them a sense of achievement. It could be when they caught their first fish, graduated from school, had a baby, or won a prize. They were asked to shut their eyes and relive the experience and then to share. This invitation to share (where they could not be accused of bragging) brought out many happy memories of jobs well done. Our ex-police chief, Bill, recalled incidents of real heroism in the line of duty. Leon had joy and sadness to share about his retirement dinner. Hazel, to our amazement, now almost incapacitated with arthritis, told about her experience as a pilot and flying instructor in World War I! Ambrose spoke of earning a $100 pay check during the Depression. From there, we spoke of the value of reminiscence, and assignments geared to Life Review seemed to follow. The ex-police chief chose humorous boyhood incidents to relate, another a family history for her grandchildren, another a religious experience.

After we had established ourselves positively in the group, we went through some sentence completion games such as:

"I'm happy when. . . ."
"I'm angry when. . . ."
"I'm scared when. . . ."
"I'm proud when. . . ."

Another opener was:

"Two things I like to do are. . . ."
"One thing that depresses me is. . . ."

If there were new members, we would go into dyads or triads and then introduce our partners, since new people had trouble relating to the entire group and felt more comfortable talking with just one or two other persons, and talking about someone other than themselves with the group as a whole. When we were at our most cohesive we would go around the group taking turns. When the group seemed ready for more insight and to take a deeper look at their own part in their problem and to take more responsibility, we tried:

"What do I do to make myself happy?"
"What do I do to make myself depressed?"

and made long lists on the blackboard. We also had fun playing the "reunion game," pretending that it was five years hence and that we were having a reunion, bragging about what we had been doing during the past five years.

We found that creative self-assignments served as antidotes to depression. For example, Fran's bragging that she had lost thirty pounds resulted in her assigning herself to go to Weight Watchers the next week instead of continuing to procrastinate. Ambrose held forth about winning golf tournaments. He hadn't played since moving to a retirement community, but with prompting from the group, he accepted an assignment to locate and try out a local golf course. Helen's report of an autobiographical family history that she planned to write as a gift to her family gave the group the perfect opportunity to encourage her to get going, and she began to write diligently.

After confirming the assignments for the following week, if there was time, we sometimes closed with the "warm fuzzy" exercise. Warm fuzzies are compliments. It is considered assertive to be able to ask for, give, and receive compliments without apologizing or overexplaining. Each member would ask anyone in the room, including the leader, for a warm fuzzy. Although some were reluctant to ask, no one ever refused to give one; these simple interchanges had a strong positive impact on both group cohesion and the self-esteem of the members.

Case Examples

Leon. Initially, Leon came in shyly and gave indications of being very depressed. He showed his last business card to his partner in a dyad during an opener and explained he had taught preretirement counseling in a large corporation, then had been forced to retire himself. When he said, softly, that he really shouldn't be depressed because he was supposed to have the answers, his eyes teared. He couldn't bring himself to speak of things he liked about himself in the present. He liked that he "used to be"—successful and a good chess player. He wasn't getting along with his wife, who was older but had much more energy than he. He was sure it was his fault and since they had just moved to this area, he had no friends. In sentence completion he said: "I'm happy when I visit with old friends. I'm not angry—I'm scared when I think of the future. . . . I'm proud of what I was." Two things he liked to do were to play chess and to read. He would like to be part of a discussion group. One thing that depressed him was inactivity and being alone too much. His assignments were to try to locate a chess partner and to make inquiries about joining a discussion group. He accepted these assignments and finally smiled when he was able to report them successfully completed. Later there were role-playing scenes illustrating a wide variety of ways one can approach one's spouse regarding marriage counseling. Since participants could volunteer to demonstrate passive ways and aggressive ways as well as assertive ones, the simulated pouting, whining, and threatening were cause for some hilarity. Leon responded to the support and positive feedback by "blossoming right before our eyes," as one member stated it. Leon became less dependent upon his wife's approval, less lonely, more active and involved in his new community.

Lola. Lola came on much stronger in the beginning. She shared during the achievement exercise that she had had her own dressmaking business when it was unusual for a woman to be that independent. Now she was retired with an adequate income and in good health. Her self-concept was that of a successful, assertive woman, both in the past and in the present. It took the openers to help her, along with the encouragement of the group, to clarify where she was afraid to be assertive. She was fearful of losing her eyesight and could not bring herself to pin the doctor down to get specific information about her condition. She felt intimidated by him and afraid of what he might say. She vacillated between aggressively denying her fears by stating she was not one to feel sorry for herself or to keep running to the doctor on the one hand, and passively withdrawing and becoming overwhelmed by her fear on the other hand. After the members role-played a wide variety of assertive approaches to the doctor, which she, in turn, rehearsed, she returned to the group to report her triumph: When the doctor had been about to finish their session and was walking out the door, she had raised her hand imperiously and said, "*Just a minute*—I am not finished." She then proceeded to read out her rehearsed questions from her notes printed in large letters. Her amazement at his attention and the thoughtfulness of his responses had been so satisfying to her that it was hard to know which had pleased her more—the assertive communication or the content of his replies.

Commentary. Assertive communication is always equal-to-equal, or in transactional analysis terms, adult-to-adult, and when aged patients allow themselves to become intimidated, they almost invite an aggressive, controlling, or indifferent response. Most doctors do an excellent job, but there are still many who appear to subscribe to the theory that old bodies are supposed to wear out and, therefore, not much can be done (Comfort, 1976). Dr. Comfort advises the elderly to be suspicious if they are told that ill health is what they can expect at their age. The group delighted in the classic assertive response that Comfort writes about from a 104-year-old man. This patient, when he complained of a stiff right knee, was told that, after all, he was 104 and couldn't expect to be agile. The old man replied, "My left knee's 104 too and it doesn't hurt!"

Bill and Elaine. Bill and Elaine were a devoted couple. Bill was the indigenous leader and self-appointed gracious host of the group. He took care of Elaine, who had multiple physical problems. Their being in the same group may well have been inhibiting to them, as they were very solicitous of each other and found it hard to express any mutual resentments in front of a group. No matter how accepting the group might have been, to do so would have been against their sense of loyalty. Their feedback was positive and perceptive and for Bill, the group obviously met his need for a feeling of importance. He clearly had some leadership skills. He had served well as a police chief in a large city. His activity had been curtailed because of both his and his wife's incapacities. But he had also lost prestige, power, and excitement in his life. In a small but important way, the group filled a little of this vacuum. He recruited members, followed up on absentees, and did so much of the "scut work" that the positive feedback Bill received, especially from the leader, was very genuine.

Elaine tended to put herself down for not being able to do the things she had been able to do before her strokes. Giving herself tiny assignments commensurate with her physical capacities and then getting massive reinforcement from the group for each new venture "shaped" or built her self-confidence along with her physical skills. Such skills included arranging flowers, making a pie (with Bill's help), then making the bed and sewing. When she was able to lose some weight and make herself a new suit, she seemed like a new person.

There was a couple who played bingo weekly in the same group as Bill and Elaine. Elaine reported with great pride that she had been very assertive with Donna. Donna had complained repeatedly that her husband, Albert, was doing a poor job at calling the numbers. Elaine had said to Donna, "If you don't care for the way Albert does it, why don't you volunteer to do it yourself?" (The group applauded.) Donna had not complained since and Elaine said it was such a relief. Now she realized that the reason she had been afraid to speak up before was because she was afraid it would come out aggressively. She explained that she no longer felt that she had to "keep the lid on," because with the help of the group, she could figure out assertive ways to express herself. There was some feeling that she spoke her mind to Bill a little more, too, but this was not dealt with directly.

Dealing with Put-Downs

Members were encouraged to share the put-downs that they had experienced or were anticipating, and then the group modeled countering them. The danger of buying into the ageist point of view that older is somehow lesser and the importance of questioning it whenever it comes up were stressed. Comfort's "bloody-mindedness" was put forth as one alternative. He feels that ageism, like racism, needs to be met by information, contradiction, and, when necessary, confrontation. And, he states, the people who are being victimized by ageism have to stand up for themselves in order to put it down.

Some of the concepts of psychological self-defense that were developed by Dr. Irene Dempsey of Davis, California, are also applicable to assertive training with the aged. According to Dr. Dempsey, there are several levels of assertiveness, starting with a total lack of awareness even of the fact that one is being put down. Next there may be a later awareness, then awareness at the time the put-down is received, but immobilization of any capacity to deal with it. Defensiveness is not as skillful as an assertive rejoinder, but superior to lack of awareness or immobilization. At least one is aware when aggression has occurred and is attempting to stand up for oneself. Counteraggression is seen here (as with Comfort) as a necessary stage of skill development in acting in one's own behalf. A humorous response represents a very high level of skill, as both parties come out unscathed. However, in learning skill in psychological self-defense, one must practice, and this may mean some counteraggression.

Choice was stressed over and over again in the group. The only choice many people know is between passively ignoring and evading a put-down or being bloody-mindedly and ragingly aggressive—either of which is usually a bad choice. But we learn that one can choose to be assertive, and there is a wide range of possible behaviors in that category from which to choose.

Some assignments that grew out of those units of learning had to do with social actions, such as writing letters to the editor or inviting a City Councilperson to speak and answer questions. Other assignments were more on a personal level, for example, a grandmother telling a daughter that she was unable to babysit, and a son that she was not too old to drive at night. The group seemed to appreciate that the concept of assertiveness meant they had more behavioral options. This carried over to many areas of their lives—from the bingo table to the doctor's office.

There is still another kind of put-down to be countered—what Comfort calls left-handed compliments. He quotes an aunt of his as saying, "The next idiot who calls me a wonderful old lady, I shall clobber." The Self-Esteem Group called it "reverse-prejudice" and compared it to statements like, "She's very intelligent, for a woman." One woman, in explaining why she found this overpraise so galling, said she almost expected to overhear someone say of her, "She's the most *remarkable* old lady. She's 69 years old and she brushes her own teeth, isn't that remarkable!" She said she'd like to counter such statements with something sarcastic, like, "He is only 26 years old and he earns his own living and has a girl-friend, isn't that remarkable!"

Conclusions

Assertive training appears to be a treatment of choice for aging people suffering losses and depression. If the depression is the result of a drop in reinforcers, a group can be a transitional step from withdrawal to building a new social network. If depression is interpreted as anger turned inward, assertive training can help the depressed person to direct his anger less destructively and more appropriately. If Otto Rank's definition of depression as being blocked creativity is applied, skill in assertive communication can lead to unblocking that creativity in the elderly.

Running a Self-Esteem Group at a meal site did not overcome the problem of irregular attendance, as had been hoped. However, the feedback from those seniors who did participate, no matter how irregularly, was positive. As the size of our aging population increases, there will be greater numbers of elderly people who develop symptoms of depression and who will not reach out for help. On the basis of self-report, completed assignments, and leader-observation, it can be concluded that this format, combining awareness and self-esteem-raising exercises with assertive training, is a viable one that warrants further development. Practicing more assertive skills in a group situation leads to the integration of those skills into the participants' repertoires of behavior, thus making it possible for them to be used more effectively as social tools in the improvement of relationships outside the group. This, in turn, is an antidote to self-limiting internalized stereotypes and low self-esteem.

Recommended Readings

Alberti, R. and Emmons, M. *Your perfect right—a guide to assertive behavior.* San Luis Obispo, CA: Impace, 1970.

Butler, R. N. and Lewis, M. I. *Aging and mental health: positive psychosocial approaches.* St. Louis, MO: C. V. Mosby, 2nd ed., 1977.

Comfort, A. *A good age.* New York: Simon and Schuster, 1976.

Corby, N. Assertive training with aged populations. *Counseling Psychologist,* 1975, *6,* #4.

Liberman, R. P. *Personal effectiveness: guiding people to assert themselves and improve their social skills.* Champaign, IL: Research Press, 1975.

Sarton, M. *Plant dreaming deep.* New York: W. W. Norton, 1968.

Schwartz, A. N. *Survival handbook for children of aging parents.* Chicago: Follett, 1977.

Silverstone, B. and Hyman, H. K. *You and your aging parent: the modern family's guide to emotional, physical and financial problems.* New York: Pantheon, 1976.

Tournier, P. *Learn to grow old.* New York: Harper and Row, 1972.

2

The Value of Widows' Groups and Emeritus Classes

Helen Kitzinger

Because of the rapid social changes in our present-day society, it is often difficult for older people to adjust to the patterns of living, which are vastly different from what they experienced when they were growing up and were part of the working world. Consequently, they are affected with more than customary stress, with loneliness, and often with physical illness.

They do not readily seek help for these problems because therapy is an alien, unknown field to them which has only recently been developed and publicized. In addition, they feel rejected by a society which tends to relegate them to a role of unimportance in our communities.

Society can therefore be said to be largely responsible for the older peoples' realistic feelings of being rejected, useless, unwanted, and unable to obtain employment. Mandatory retirement and being out of the work force lowers not only their self-esteem but their income. Inflation has forced them often to sell their own homes and to live in inferior housing, subjecting them to a generally lower standard of living. They often suffer from poor nutrition, and their health insurance is inadequate to cover medical needs.

Until some relief in these areas can be obtained, we cannot expect older people voluntarily to seek counseling or therapy, especially with the threat of greater expense and the additional problem of transportation. Understandably, their feeling is, "What's the use? I'm too old anyway."

Many older people are fearful of trying out new projects and meeting new challenges. They feel inadequate, become lonely and depressed. They fear their families will place them in a nursing home. Often they use alcohol and drugs to lessen their loneliness and to enable them to sleep. They try in this way to avoid anxiety and depression. Ever present is the fear of incapacitating illness. Many become hypercritical of their relatives and families, expecting more help and attention than can reasonably be given, failing to realize that sons and daughters may need to work and have responsibilities for their own children.

On the other hand, of course, many of the activities undertaken by older people have indirect therapeutic benefits. Volunteer work with community agencies falls in this category: helping the handicapped, chatting with or shopping for people in nursing or retirement homes, visiting hospital patients or selling in the gift shop. As a member of Senior Companion Services the older person might visit the homebound—comparable to themselves in age—to deliver library books, shop for groceries, and provide an all-around atmosphere of companionship and caring. This raises the morale of both receiver and giver.

Or the older person might become active in Senior Citizen Centers where one can meet others to play bridge or checkers, learn square dancing, join discussion groups, and participate in many other activities. Just establishing communication with others can be of tremendous benefit, alleviating loneliness, maintaining interest in the community, and often heading off placement in a nursing home. However, such associations, valuable as they may be, are not likely to compensate for major losses suffered by older people, notably the death of a spouse.

A Group for the Widowed

One good-sized segment of older people that has been more or less ignored until recently consists of widows and widowers. Widowed persons suddenly find themselves grief-stricken and alone without a partner, having to make many decisions on problems with which they have never before been confronted. Their life-style is completely changed. Should they continue to live in the same house or apartment where they have been living or should they seek a new location? Should they live with a friend, or a son or daughter? Will their finances be severely curtailed, and if so, what do they do about this problem? These and many more personal questions present themselves and cause added grief and confusion.

In order to try to offset some of the stress and grief following the death of a spouse, the writer formed, some four years ago, a group of recently bereaved men and women. After the leader had arranged with one of the community agencies for weekly use of a room at no charge, the local paper agreed to publicize the new group in its section on community activities. A signed article stressing the loneliness of widowhood announced that a group was being formed, led by a psychologist, where widows and widowers could discuss cooperatively the problems resulting from the death of their spouses. Interested people were asked to call, and individual interviews were arranged so the purpose of the group could be explained and each person's interest in participating could be determined.

Nine women and five men were accepted, and attendance at the meetings turned out to be fairly regular. As a rule, when outside commitments prevented members from attending a session, they either informed the leader or notified her through another of the participants. On the whole, members were serious and intent upon working through problems evolving from their new single status. Mutual help and support were given. There was a friendly interchange of ideas and comments between men and women, with no attempt at dating one another or playing up to the opposite sex.

The group started out rather dramatically. Two women came crying to the first session and upon entering the room loudly threatened suicide. The group had formed a circle with their chairs. These two were invited to join this circle, but pulled their chairs away and sat behind the others. They did not participate verbally. At the second session they entered the room and voluntarily joined the circle but remained silent. In succeeding sessions they gradually were able to express feeling, no longer mentioning suicide. Later they referred to it as an urge in the past. They gradually became accepted members of the group, earning their acceptance through participation, sometimes active, sometimes passive.

All were encouraged in the group setting to express their feelings, their pain, their love, and their dependency needs as well as their grief. Crying was condoned as a recognized need and as an expression of their own mourning, their shock, frustration, and anger at their present unwelcome and unforeseen new circumstances of living.

The normal reactions to sudden loss of a spouse were explained as: (1) shock and disbelief; (2) crying and blaming doctors, nurses, family members for possible causes of death; (3) mourning in which the reality of death is finally recognized; (4) obsession with thoughts of the person, memories recalled until the image of the dead person becomes devoid of negative undesirable features; (5) the healing process which may take months or weeks; (6) the final ability to move forward and make constructive plans (Taves, 1968).

After grief was somewhat assuaged, loneliness and depression became the primary complaints. The leader suggested several ways of handling these: seeking activities at the agency and in the community, talking to a close friend, finding new hobbies, taking courses at Emeritus College, signing up for volunteer work, or helping friends and neighbors in need. But the responsibility for finding an acceptable solution or plan that best suited their needs was placed upon the individual members.

The members were encouraged to describe how they had managed to cope with this problem up to the present, though it was generally admitted that no completely satisfactory solutions would be found. However, finding others in the group with similar interests and needs for friendship was a definite step in making contacts with one another and reaching out beyond themselves for new relationships and activities.

There was one woman in the group who, because of traumatic experiences accompanying the death of her husband and her son, seemed unable to move forward in activity of any kind. She spoke very little in the group and could not be drawn out by either the others or the leader. Subsequently, she was referred by the leader to an agency for individual counseling. This agency offered her a clerical job in their office where she continued working contentedly.

Interest in the group kept up for three or four months, though one or two of the members dropped out. One became ill; another got married to someone outside the group.

For those who stayed, however, the improvement was noticeable. For one thing, they were dealing more realistically with their feelings. For example, two or three withdrawn people were able to talk about their depression and, even more significant, their anger. Many were seeing each other socially on weekends, taking walks together, attending concerts or eating together. The widows tended to meet together. This was especially true for one small group of four, who seemed to become close friends. Evidence of this was manifest in discussions of a social nature such as arranging for outings, picnics, and even two- or three-day bus trips to places of interest.

At the end of about four months the leader felt it was no longer necessary to meet on a regular basis since all seemed to be managing and felt that they had talked out their problems.

Case Examples

Marian. On joining the group, Marian, widowed about eight years and then about 55 years of age, lived with her married daughter, who had two children. Marian acted as a babysitter, when needed, but had no car of her own, so needed to borrow her daughter's in order to go out anywhere. She was able to express her dissatisfaction with the total subservience to her daughter, and her unhappy life in general.

Group was understanding and helped her make decisions to form a new life for herself independent of her daughter. First, she canceled a summer trip to France, where she was to go to see relatives. With the money she would have spent on this trip, she rented a small apartment, bought a second-hand car, and thus achieved independence and self-reliance. She was able to get a part-time job and expressed feelings of satisfaction and contentment with her new way of living.

Bertha. Bertha, 57 years of age, recently widowed, came to the group crying, threatening suicide, and said she had no wish to live. She complained of loneliness and no friends. For the first two sessions, she sat apart from the group (as previously mentioned) and did not participate in discussions. Finally, she moved her chair into the circle, participated in group discussions, and, after the third session, stopped crying and seemed almost cheerful. The leader arranged for her to do volunteer work after she said she needed something to keep her busy. She began to work four days a week as a volunteer, three at the United Nations office and one with Travelers Aid at the airport. She also obtained some paid part-time work, selling jewelry at a department store. Later she booked passage for a month's tour alone, visiting parts of Europe and Russia. On her return she resumed all of her volunteer work plus some paid part-time selling.

Herbert. In contrast to these two women was a 63-year-old widower who seemed to gain little or no therapeutic benefit from the group. He started out by stating at the first session that the group was not for him—he didn't like it. However, he did not leave and attended regularly. When the discussion touched on any kind of grief, he left the room, returning after a few minutes and explaining that the subject did not interest him. He became overfriendly with some of the women, holding their hands, putting his arm around them, and sitting as close to them as possible. (It was difficult to know whether they enjoyed this kind of physical contact or merely tolerated it, but none of the women expressed disapproval.) He had no insight into his problems and shortcomings, but the leader decided not to exclude him, though his presence sometimes interfered with the progress of the group. After the group ceased to meet, he continued with the informal gatherings.

Subsequent Groups for the Widowed

Second Group

Formation of a second group was arranged at the same center about six months later. A notice was again placed in the local paper, but no individual interviews were held. About eight widows appeared for the first meeting and expressed extreme disappointment that no widowers had come. Their dress and appearance showed that they had taken more than usual care to look as attractive as possible. They showed obvious disinterest in listening to anyone else's pain or grief but were intent only on talking about themselves and the crisis in which they suddenly found themselves. No interchange of feeling took place, and the leader wondered how progress could be made on the basis of their egocentricity and lack of interest in the problems of others.

As an example of the attitudes in this group, and of the disinterest in the objectives expressed by the leader, the following case may be cited:

Case Example

Selma Selma, a slim, rather unattractive 58-year-old widow, expressed no particular grief for the recent demise of her husband but was intent on telling the other members of the group how well she was making the adjustment. Her method was to advertise in the local paper for a male boarder to take into her home. She said she always made interrogations about his financial state, and if it was good, accepted him. Group members informed her what a dangerous procedure this could be. She refused to listen and went on to say that in addition she drank all evening, as this enabled her to sleep with the addition of a sleeping pill. She expressed much satisfaction with this solution to living alone and said since she was happy, she had no intention of making any changes.

Although obviously some individual counseling or therapy was indicated and was suggested to her, she became hostile and saw no need for it.

Commentary. It was interesting to the leader that though others in the group saw the danger in admitting a man into her home without careful scrutiny of his credentials, they seemed not to question her escape from loneliness via liquor and sleeping pills.

As it happened, none returned for the second meeting. One member of this group, however, telephoned the leader to say she needed friends and would like to make a date for lunch. The leader explained that the pressure of work was such that an immediate appointment would be impossible but that if this member would call the following week an appointment could be arranged. Apparently she was frustrated in her attempt to see the leader alone; she did not phone again.

Third Group

At the second session an entirely new group of seven widows appeared. Their behavior and lack of empathy duplicated the events of the previous meeting. Two women departed abruptly in mid-session and the others at the end; no attempt was made to communicate with the leader. A third meeting was not held.

Despite her unfortunate experience with the last group, the leader was receptive when an agency in Beverly Hills expressed interest in having her start their own group for widows. The agency recruited people and explained the purpose of the meetings. Six widows, ranging in age from 36 to 65 (but mostly over 50), came to the sessions, all eager to participate.

The problems were varied. One young widow whose husband had suddenly committed suicide was distraught by the problems of caring for her children. The group was supportive and helpful, encouraging her to continue the law studies which she had begun a few years previously. In a second case, an older woman complained that she mostly served as a babysitter for her eight-year-old grandson and also as the dog-walker for her daughter's family when they went away on trips. The group aided her in understanding that she felt too guilty about her resentment toward her daughter to be able to express her true feelings. With the help of the other women in the group, she became more aware of her own feelings and came to feel confident that in the future she would be able to handle the daughter's frequent demands on her time.

In this same group one widow stands out as having had the most traumatic experiences of all. During the previous year her mother and twin brother in England had both died, and her own husband, to whom she was devoted, died unexpectedly. Then her 30-year-old married daughter with three young children died of cancer. This was too much: the widow attempted suicide via sleeping pills, but a son discovered her and she recovered after a few days in the hospital.

During the first few sessions she was understandably distraught, but the group members were most helpful with their sympathy and understanding. She began to make plans: to see her grandchildren whenever possible, to take classes to improve her physical condition and health, to occupy herself with reading. She decided to remain in her own home rather than move. Altogether she was realistic and began to adjust well to her new life situation.

After the group disbanded she remained in telephone contact with the leader. That fall Emeritus College classes began in Santa Monica. She immediately signed up for the leader's class and has continued to attend classes regularly. She also enrolled for other courses and is interested in continuing to learn and to socialize with the people she meets. She informed the leader recently that her late daughter's husband has now remarried, and though not particularly fond of his new wife, she is managing to face this problem and keep in contact with her grandchildren.

After meeting for approximately ten sessions, the group had to be terminated because the summer months arrived and most of the members would be going away on vacation. In summary, the group members had helped each other either to alter their life patterns to conform with present needs or to become aware of changes in their life-styles which would be necessary in the future.

Overview of Widowed Groups

A major theme stressed by the leader in all groups was the need to reassess one's life. Looking back over the topics discussed, and the attitudes and behavior shown by the group members, she concludes that much more change occurred in some areas than in others. For example, the expression of grief by a member and its acceptance by the others seemed definitely to aid the process of bereavement and in the long run to reduce depression. Several of the widows learned to cope better with loneliness, whether through becoming more adept at initiating social contacts, through undertaking new activities, or simply through becoming more comfortable in the new role of a single person. It seemed to the leader that decreasing dependence upon alcohol and drugs was shown by some of the group members, at least during the time the leader was with the group. Two or three of the group members showed evidence of becoming more assertive in dealing with requests and demands made by their children and other family members.

On the other hand, the leader failed to note any perceptible change in dealing with other problems, such as jealousy, living alone, fear of crime and of going out at night, or fear of illness and ultimately having to enter a nursing home.

In general, though with some exceptions, it seems fair to say that the widows' group experience at least partially restored the members' self-esteem and confidence, helped them make new friends, and encouraged their reaching for new interests and involvements, leading to their reintegration into the community. Thus, the will to live seemed definitely reestablished.

Emeritus College Classes

Certain Emeritus College classes are another setting in which nontraditional therapy with older people takes place. In 1975 Santa Monica College became one of the first to establish an emeritus college program primarily for the 20,000 residents of the city of Santa Monica who are 60 years of age or older, most of them retired and a few homebound.

Several community colleges in various parts of the United States have set up emeritus programs, a few of them being sufficiently well organized to be called "emeritus colleges." These programs are specifically designed to meet the needs of older persons. Their classes are held only during the daytime, minimal or no fees are charged, and a wide variety of study subjects is offered. The general aim is to encourage older persons to expand their horizons, become more interested in their surroundings, and communicate more meaningfully with people of all ages. Emeritus classes are essentially for persons who are active and eager to become involved with new ideas. They are designed to challenge and appeal to the older individual whose interests may have become limited or confined to a small group of friends. For some, life has become dull. For people in this

Older Women Practice Creative Living

Lillian Kratz is a specialist in counseling and teaching older adults, and a supervisor of peer counselors at Andrus Gerontology Center. For UCLA Extension she prepared a course, "Creative Living," for women between 50 and the late 70s, an age at which they often feel trapped by the stereotyped roles into which society has placed them. In lectures and both large and small group discussions, they examine the myths and stereotypes and explore the changing of roles at this stage of life, the increase of self-awareness and improvement of interpersonal relationships.

Ms. Kratz stresses that before changing roles or goals one must know what kind of person she is. So the class members fill out a "Hierarchy of Values" questionnaire and discuss it in small groups, obtaining significant feedback on their ability to change. An item is chosen from a list of individual and personal problems submitted to the leader at the start of each class. The problem relates to the day's topic and is the basis for group discussion, which often becomes group therapy, with insights and shared reactions growing out of a supportive atmosphere.

Betty, age 62, one of the class members, defined her problem thus: "I can't seem to attract people. I like them but they don't warm up to me. It's even happening in this class. I've always had some of this problem, but it seems much worse now."

She was asked to participate in two exercises on "how you come across to others." Working with a small group of four, she got feedback on the discrepancy between her verbal and nonverbal behavior and on her failure to listen to others. In the full group she was able to perceive that she, who liked people, came across as a cold person. She stated it with insight: "They think I'm cool because I *act* cool."

Betty continued in the next Kratz class, evidencing good awareness of the discrepancy between what she wanted to convey and what she was portraying. With much positive reinforcement from both leader and class, she made notable progress in expressing herself warmly and attractively to others, which produced greater confidence in herself and in her ability to relate to others.

situation the classes offer new stimulation, new friends, and the opportunity for intellectual and emotional growth.

In Santa Monica, Emeritus College classes are held in about twenty-five different locations in the city (churches, banks, community centers, etc.), thereby easing the transportation problem. Classes are offered in more than fifty subjects, including art, languages and culture, health, history, literature, current events, music, philosophy, and psychology. Many people enroll for more than one course. Sessions are generally two hours in length, including a short intermission. During this time students socialize or discuss scholarly or personal problems with each other and often with the instructor.

Emeritus classes are not given for credit, and there are no academic requirements for enrollment. This gives the instructor much more leeway than in regular college or university classes, and makes it possible to guide the course in a therapeutic direction. For example, in the class called "Psychosocial Trends in a Changing Society," the instructor stimulated the sharing of views on the facts and myths of aging, the meaning of retirement, changing family relationships, and community facilities for volunteer work. Other subjects which came up for discussion in this class were loneliness, depression, stress, drugs and alcohol, nutrition, and crime. It was not necessary to encourage the airing of personal problems; the subject matter and the permissive setting induced it. In one lively discussion the members of the class spoke of problems with their grown children and their families. They decided they tended to make excessive demands on their married children, expecting far more attention and time from them than was realistic.

Among the subjects most frequently discussed were living on fixed incomes amid the inroads of inflation, high medical fees, and fear of illness and placement in nursing homes. The class seemed to be helped by feeling that all older people face similar problems. Although specific solutions were seldom found, the feeling that they could verbalize these concerns enabled the members to concentrate on more positive activities.

As might be expected, some courses are especially adapted to bringing about personal and therapeutic benefits. For example, "Interpersonal Relationships," "Stress Reduction," "Healthful Living," "Personal Growth," and "Human Potential Regardless of Age," are courses of this type which have all been given recently in the Emeritus College. Several of the instructors have commented on various signs of an improved general outlook on living which they have noted in their students.

Possibly a more valuable source of information is the students themselves. The Emeritus College Research Committee sent out a questionnaire to over 600 class members to discover whether their needs were being met. In general they were; ratings on teaching proficiency and on class discussion and atmosphere were affirmative and enthusiastic. More interesting from our standpoint were their comments about the changes they saw in themselves as a result of the classroom experiences. Here are several excerpts:

> I have discovered my capability to do things which I had no time to pursue in younger years. I have met wonderful people who became my friends. Emeritus College and its courses have given me self-confidence. (A 65-plus-year-old former office worker, living with her husband.)

> I have a better self-image since I am combining work with play. It's fun as well as informative. (An under-55-year-old with no post-high school attendance.)

> I look forward to attending classes to apply what is learned to relieve stress and feel hopeful instead of helpless; to be one of a group and share the same interests; to enlarge my horizons; I am enriching my life. (A 70-plus-year-old living alone, with no previous college education.)

> It really has helped me greatly. I've come out of my shell. Can't say enough for it! (An under-55-year-old homemaker.)

> The College has taken me out of myself—given me not only more knowledge but more self-esteem and confidence. Before attending various classes, I had been ill, immobile, depressed for many years. I am grateful to have this privilege. I would be lost without Emeritus. (A 70-plus-year-old with no previous post-high school education.)

> I believe Emeritus College is one of the most positive programs offered to the Senior. It exercises not only the physical but also the "mental muscle" as well. It gives people on low income a chance to associate with people of similar interests. I have seen people who have sat home depressed; after a writing class or something they had never tried before they found new abilities and became different people. We should thank God every day for these classes and the dedicated, beautiful teachers that have given us understanding, friendship, encouragement. (A 70-plus-year-old, living alone, with no previous college education.)

Many of the Emeritus College programs contain courses with therapeutic value for seniors. For example, the Emeritus Institute of Saddleback College in Mission Viejo (Orange County), California, has classes in

- Fundamentals of aging
- Health and happiness in the later years

- Being a grandparent
- Assertive skills
- Reach out/volunteerism
- Horizons for widows and widowers

Similar opportunities for enrichment and growth are offered in the Bay Area—e.g., the Emeritus Institute of Cañada College in Redwood City and the Emeritus College of Marin in Kentfield, California. The American Association for Community and Junior Colleges in Washington tries to keep up with the rapidly expanding programs for older people and can give information about resources in any part of the country (address of the AACJC: 1 Dupont Circle, N.W., Washington, D.C. 20036).

Recommended Readings

Edwards, M. and Hoover, E. *The challenge of being single.* Los Angeles: Tarcher, 1974.

Morse, T. *Life is for living.* Garden City, NY: Doubleday, 1973.

Peterson, J. and Briley, M. *Widows and widowhood.* New York: Association Press, 1977.

Taves, I. *Women alone.* New York: Funk and Wagnalls, 1968.

Block, J. L. *Back in circulation.* New York: Macmillan, 1969.

Curtin, S. R. *Nobody ever died of old age.* Boston: Little, Brown, 1972.

Hendin, D. *Death as a fact of life.* New York: Norton, 1973.

Kline, N. *From sad to glad.* New York: Putnam, 1974.

3

Adult Day-Care Centers: A Potent Force for Individual and Family Change

Lynn Leonard

Because adult day care is still a relatively new service in the United States, many of us who work in this area have been more than a little dazzled by the novelty of the setting and the image of ourselves as pioneers. Fortunately, our clients, the "frail" elderly, have confronted us with their startling capacity for growth and change. As a result, we as helping professionals and paraprofessionals have been jolted out of our comfortable caregiver roles and are delighted to discover ourselves now actively engaged in dynamic, growth-enhancing relationships with persons who were previously in danger of passing through the nursing home door to the isolation and quiet desperation beyond.

In this chapter I will share with you what we have learned from participants in adult day-care programs which are sponsored in the Greater Phoenix Metropolitan area by the Foundation for Senior Adult Living, Inc. (FSAL). The first part of this chapter is devoted to a description of approaches we have found useful in reducing the threat that counseling holds for frail older persons who participate in adult day-care centers as an alternative to nursing-home placement. In these centers, older persons receive the daytime care and supervision which permits them to remain in their own homes or with their families. In the remainder of the chapter, I will be describing some of the ways in which we have attempted to work with the families of our participants. Those of us who work in our agency's day-care programs have been amazed at the gains our participants can make when we are truly attuned to them and their families. We have discovered that our programs can be much more than a means for preventing premature institutionalization of frail older persons. When we function as an effective team, the adult day-care center becomes a natural setting and potent agent for therapeutic gain for the entire family.

Finding the Nonthreatening Approach

One of the first lessons our participants taught us was that our sense of timing was off. We were either in too great a hurry to "establish rapport," or we were too quick to conclude that "rapport would be difficult, if not impossible to establish due to advanced organic brain syndrome." Those of us who had been trained as counselors or as members of some other "talking" profession were the slowest learners. We were accustomed to establishing trust by verbal means. It took us a while to realize that what participants do and how they do it may be vastly more significant than what they say to us during our first two or three chats with them. We had forgotten that the people we were trying to work with belonged to a generation that holds dear the conviction that "deeds speak louder than words"!

Case Example

Mrs. Jones. Mrs. Jones brought this first lesson home to us. At 75, Mrs. Jones had been a widow for fourteen months when she first came to the Center after moving to Phoenix six months earlier to live with her daughter and son-in-law. In New York she had become a prisoner in her apartment, trapped there by cold, snow, and the fear of muggers. At the Center, it was reported during her case conference, Mrs. Jones talked only of her plans to return to New York after her hip had completely healed from corrective surgery. In the weekly group sessions with other widows, the social worker noted that Mrs. Jones "expressed no feelings relative to the loss of her husband." Activity personnel expressed concern that Mrs. Jones threw the ball too vigorously to other participants during the exercise program, and the Center Director noted that Mrs. Jones was "playful" and sometimes used her cane to hook the ankle of staff members as they passed by.

A social work student became interested in Mrs. Jones after Mrs. Jones had literally "hooked" her attention with the cane. After the exercise class one morning, Mary, the student, commented on Mrs. Jones's strong throwing arm and excellent aim. She invited Mrs. Jones out into the yard where there was more room and less danger of an accident. They talked while throwing the ball, and Mrs. Jones began to express her anger toward her husband for "the trick he played on me by dying first."

Mrs. Jones and Mary developed a twice-weekly routine of "catch" out in the yard, and as Mrs. Jones's hip grew better, they went for short walks. A few weeks later Mrs. Jones began to share in group with the other widows those thoughts she had expressed and found accepted during the "catch" sessions and walks with Mary.

During their first case conference concerning Mrs. Jones, staff identified her anger and attention-seeking behaviors and explored the motivation for them. Initially, staff felt they had failed to establish rapport, but as they continued to share their observations of Mrs. Jones, they noted that she "hooked" only staff with her cane, never other participants. Staff concluded this behavior might indicate that her attention-seeking was directed toward those whom she appropriately perceived to be in a helping role. Clearly, Mrs. Jones was a person whose actions, rather than words, were indicative of her true feelings.

Had staff failed to accurately read Mrs. Jones's behavior (which would likely have happened without the structure of the case conference) and had staff instead insisted Mrs. Jones respond on a verbal level in the group sessions, one wonders whether Mrs. Jones would ever have had the opportunity to express her feelings and find acceptance for them from staff, peers, and, finally, from within herself.

Commentary. Older persons' general discomfort in discussing feelings is, we feel, a given in therapeutic endeavors with the elderly. Once this is acknowledged as natural for them, then many means can be devised and employed for working around the "resistance."

For instance, in our centers we have observed that discussions about feelings seem to occur naturally and more readily when three or four older persons are sitting around a table, each engaged in his or her own handiwork or crafts project. After the community singalong one afternoon, I joined four ladies at a table, all of whom were crocheting, engrossed in conversation while waiting for the Center van to come to take them home. Each smiled and acknowledged my presence, but continued to crochet. The conversation also resumed. Erma told Arliss, "I wish I felt the way you do, but I'm afraid to die. My mother had a real dread of it. I think that's why she was so crazy the last six years of her life." Arliss responded, "I used to feel that way, scared and all. But now, it seems kind of natural. I mean, think how terrible it would be if no one ever died, if we had no choice but to live forever and ever. I don't know, but I think the idea of living on and on and on is a lot scarier than dying."

After this incident, the staff at the Center decided that our usual schedule of group discussion followed by crafts might not be the best approach. Instead, the group leader began to join the ladies at their end of the table for "chat time." This has worked out quite well and sometimes as many as ten older persons, men and women, contribute to discussions that have ranged in topic from "death or dying" to "how to let your grown children know that you may be old and have a little trouble getting around, but that ain't a reason to treat you like you're feeble-minded, too!" At this Center, Betty Josephson, the Health Coordinator, opted to forego a move into a new, relatively plush and private office when renovations at the Center were completed. Betty decided to keep the little 7' X 7' cubbyhole she had always used that had been temporarily partitioned off at the end of the Activity Room. She says:

> The participants can unobtrusively drop in to chat with me on their way back from the bathroom. Their peers don't notice it, and the noise outside in the Activity Area creates a feeling of privacy in here. Usually, they begin with a health problem—say a concern about their blood pressure. Usually, I think this is just a request for touch, but I check it out, as I'm taking the cuff off, the real concern usually surfaces. I do a lot of one-to-one in here. I think maybe because I'm a nurse, it seems natural to explore problems with me. Social workers and counselors have a harder time initially because not everyone here has known a social worker or counselor before, and maybe they associate social workers and counselors with people who need financial assistance or help with personal or relationship problems. These people really hate appearing in need of help in these areas.

Betty has beautifully summed up what we feel is the key to therapeutic intervention with older clients. The majority of these clients will be receptive to our therapeutic endeavors as long as we *appear* initially to be offering some other kind of assistance. The beauty of the day-care setting is that there is so much time and so many opportunities to make counseling an older person an integral but *incidental* part of the program.

Dealing with the Family Therapeutically

Similarly, our work with the families of our participants has been incidental to our education program. Our centers have invited family members to participate in evening sessions in which key staff persons—the social worker, nurse, dietitian, and occupational therapist—will share with families information that will make it easier for them to maintain their older family member in their own home.

These groups or classes, therefore, are begun on an educational, informative basis. We share useful information: how to adapt the home economically to the safety needs of a stroke patient; how to manage the proper diet for a diabetic but still please the family palate without doubling food preparation time and effort; how to assist in the transfer of a paraplegic while protecting your own back. Through these classes we convey to families that we are concerned about them, too, and that we are interested in helping them. This approach has an interesting history.

In our early work in adult day care, we realized that we were thinking and acting like the staff of many old-style child guidance centers who, tending to see children as victims, all too often acted in a punitive manner toward their parents. Of course, in our case we placed the "black hats" on the grown children who served as caretakers. At this stage in our experience, our motivation for bringing families together for sessions was usually to set the family on the right track so that they would facilitate rather than impede our therapeutic efforts with their parents or older family member. Not surprisingly, these sessions were not particularly well attended.

Interacting as we did on a daily basis with the older family member, we were far more aware of and sensitive to their pain and problems than those of their families. Naturally, but unwisely, we viewed the families with some suspicion, and we actually set up a classic situation of the self-fulfilling prophecy. "I really didn't think Mrs. Smith's daughter would be willing to invest in helping her mother and she wasn't! She came to only one of the sessions." In retrospect, we are certain Mrs. Smith's daughter *was* willing to invest or she wouldn't have come to any sessions. She simply wasn't responsive to our evangelistic, thinly veiled, "Heathen, repent!" approach!

Fortunately for everyone concerned, we soon examined our motives and attitudes and realized the trap we'd fallen into. We recalled some of the principles we'd learned in our family therapy classes. "When one person in the family is in pain, all are in pain." At this point we began to focus actively on the family unit as our primary client. Since then, our work has been far more challenging and productive.

The challenge comes from having to broaden our focus. We've had to relearn what, in our focus in gerontology, we'd forgotten about life-span psychology, developmental tasks, and their crises. In working with a three- and sometimes four-generation family, a narrow focus in gerontology is apt to fall short of the mark!

Our recent approach to families is far different. Our initial invitation to them, as stated earlier, is simple: "Let us share some tips on how to ease the load we know you're carrying." Within this context, and having experienced our staff as concerned about them and their problems, family members begin to open up to us and to the other group members, at first with problems of management, but ones which reveal some family dynamics and information for future work with the family as a unit.

Case Example

Mrs. Brown. "I get so angry with him." (Mrs. Brown is talking about her 82-year-old father, Mr. White, who has lived for five years with her, her husband and their four children, ages 5 to 17.) "He won't take a bath at all, and I have to nag to get him to shave; and when he does, he misses half his beard. He smells! Last week our teenagers told me they aren't bringing any of their friends home until I get him to take a bath. The other day he went in to bathe—at least I thought he did. I heard the water running, and he was in there for over a half hour. Finally John, our oldest, pounded on the door and when Dad didn't answer, John got scared and went on into the bathroom. Dad was just sitting and grinning, fully clothed, on the toilet. There was water in the tub, but he was just trying to make us think he'd taken a bath. John thought it was hilarious. It reminded him of what he used to do when he was about 11, and had an aversion to water."

In the course of the discussion that followed, on a practical level the installation of grab bars was recommended in order to reduce Mr. White's fear of falling. Another group member suggested that maybe John could help his grandfather shave. This seemed workable, since John had identified with his grandfather's means of coping with Mrs. Brown's nagging. The social worker made a mental note that at no time in the discussion did Mrs. Brown mention her husband or his reactions to her father.

As a result of a subsequent case conference, the social worker arranged to stop by the home to talk with Mrs. Brown some morning with a view to paving the way for Mr. and Mrs. Brown to join a planned group for couples who had a parent living with them. Mr. Brown happened to be home that day and, after some initially awkward moments, responded to the social worker's interest in him and his midlife career change and move to Arizona. She applauded Mr. Brown's courage in leaving a secure job to risk establishing himself in a new field. The invitation to join the couple's group was accepted by Mr. and Mrs. Brown, and after four weeks of participation, Center staff noted that Mr. White was neater and cleaner when he came to the Center. He also paced and wandered less and began to take an active interest in the Center. He volunteered to be the Center handyman. He fixed doors that stuck or wouldn't close, made a new mailbox, and appointed himself to keep the patio area clean and neat. His new behaviors facilitated his integration into the group. At the annual Center Christmas party, Mr. Brown told the social worker, "Things really began to improve for us after we got involved here. In a way, I guess we owe it all to Helen's Dad. You wouldn't have been helping us if he hadn't been in our home. What's funny is that I used to resent him and Helen so much. I blamed them for the fact that my big decision to uproot and try a new career at 42 was rougher than I'd thought it would be."

Commentary. When intervention is successful, as it was with the Browns, the senior citizen achieves a more positive status within the family. No longer is he viewed as an additional or causative stress agent. Instead, he is viewed as the means by which help became available to a family in trouble and in pain.

Given our focus on the entire family system and all of its members, and given our role of facilitator and family system supporter and strengthener, it has become obvious that we can in no way afford to be narrow specialists in gerontology. Our specialty must be far broader. We must be knowledgeable in the area of human development throughout the life span. We must know as much about and be as understanding of the developmental tasks and crises of adolescence as we are of the tasks and crises of old age. We must understand and be sensitive to the phenomena of the midlife crisis, the feeling that time enough does not remain to accomplish all that was planned for in early adulthood. We must be as sensitive to these developmental tasks and crises as we are to the tasks of old age, the task of reviewing one's life and declaring oneself satisfied or dissatisfied with the results.

Families will readily seek our assistance in coping with the stresses of crowding and diminished privacy, of increased financial burden, or management of generational conflict, of compelling responsibilities, and of adapting the home to accommodate the older person who experiences sensory, motor, and/or memory impairments. But we must be sensitive to what is often *unrecognized* by the family and therefore is *not verbalized to us.* Each family member copes not only with the stresses just enumerated; he or she also struggles *simultaneously* for a satisfactory resolution of his or her own developmental crisis. It is within this broad and complex context that our work with day-care participant and family must be accomplished.

Advantages of the Day-Care Setting

A considerable degree of our success in working with frail older persons is simply a result of the day-care setting. Therapeutic intervention is easier when clients are with us six hours a day, three to five days per week. Our clients—participants and their families—are naturally inclined to trust us; the participant because we prevent his institutionalization, the family because we share in the care of a disabled older person, thus relieving them of constant caretaker responsibilities or freeing both husband and wife for paid employment. In addition, our programs provide nutrition, health surveillance, transportation to and from the Center and to medical and social service appointments, and recreation and socialization. Nursing care is available at two centers and therapies (physical, speech, and occupational) are also available in varying intensities in all four adult day-care programs. The provision of tangible services that our clients experience as providing for their security and safety greatly enhances our effectiveness as we assist them in meeting their needs for information, esteem, affiliation, and actualization.

While three of our programs offer so-called maintenance or Level II day-care services and are funded through a Title XX contract which limits the amount of resources that can be aimed at medical (restorative) intervention, we have found that measurable improvement in the level of functioning is achievable to some degree with most clients. Our findings are substantiated by the increased performance our clients achieve on a Care Assessment scale we have adapted for use in our programs. This scale includes: (1) a functional assessment of the ability to perform the activities of daily living (bathing, eating, grooming, toileting, walking, etc); (2) mental status; (3) morale; and (4) socialization. Assessments are made prior to the participant's entry into the program and again at least every three months. A plan of care is developed for each participant and is amended as specific goals are achieved or as the specified approach and/or goal is found to be unworkable or unrealistic.

Because our clients are either physically disabled, mentally disoriented, or severely withdrawn and depressed, our daily activity programs are designed to facilitate improvement in each of these areas. Our interdisciplinary day-care team—social worker, nurse, activity coordinator, occupational therapist, and registered dietitian—ensure that overall program design is sound and growth-producing. Physical and speech therapists' consultation is also available to the care team.

Naturally, we feel best when our participants improve and graduate into programs such as RSVP, congregate nutrition programs, or senior center activities. Approximately 17 percent have accomplished this despite an average age of 79. Recently, four participants became Senior Companions and now receive a stipend for their services to other frail older persons!

However, nearly 70 percent of our participants remain in our day-care programs for long-term care (18 months or longer). Of this group, over 40 percent have been with us since the programs began, three or four years ago [TELOCA Center began in December 1974, El Rinconcito in April 1975, Sirrine in December 1975, and Longview (Level I Day Care) in January 1979.]. Of those leaving the program after receiving either short-term or long-term care, a surprising number (18 percent) have moved out of state, sometimes with their families, sometimes to live with other relatives. Approximately 13 percent have died while in the programs, and another 12 percent do eventually enter nursing homes, usually after another severe illness has resulted first in hospitalization. We do not view these nursing home entries as a sign of failure, however, because on an average, they participate in adult day-care for fifteen months prior to nursing-home placement. In other words, for these people, our programs have forestalled placement by an average of fifteen months.

The effectiveness of our work in adult day care is increased because our service does not stand alone. These programs are part of a network of services and facilities provided by our sponsor, the Foundation for Senior Adult Living, Inc. (FSAL) in its efforts to enrich the lives of older adults throughout the cycle of senior adult life. RSVP and Senior Adult Neighborhood Groups (SANGS) provide vol-

Therapy via the Senior Center

Abby Hellwarth is director of a southwestern urban multipurpose center for older people, whose clients are 95 percent black and 25 percent at the poverty level. She reports that the center gives them an opportunity to do things denied them in their working lives. Mrs. Johnson, for example, had been a domestic in households where the wives were engaged in charitable activities. Now out of work because of illness and depression, she was persuaded by a friend to come to the center. Here she found herself by taking over the fund-raising responsibility and becoming involved in activities she learned from her former employers. Similarly, a former cook for the school system is doing what she always wanted to do: teaching a sewing and arts and crafts class. A retired postal supervisor is doing employment counseling and publicity. These people are no longer suffering from the loss of self-confidence and self-esteem often associated with retirement.

Resistance to therapeutic efforts does, however, occur; the once a week personal counselor has found that the best way to get people to come in and talk is to announce that she is taking blood pressure—a much-desired local service!

The multipurpose center functions to some extent as a day-care center and is able to help a limited number of confused and dependent elderly persons. One widow who had been attending the center had her home broken into and mementoes of her late husband stolen. For days she could talk only about the burglary and her loss. Everyone listened and tried to reassure her, which helped greatly. Without the center she would probably have had to be institutionalized, but like many others she was able to keep going because of the psychological and social supports furnished. Mrs. Hellwarth is convinced that a multipurpose center can play an important role in keeping the functioning elderly from becoming the "frail elderly."

unteer and socialization opportunities for active and healthy older persons. Housing, much of which includes rent subsidy, is also available or planned for the active and healthy older person. Programs and facilities for seniors who need limited care and/or rehabilitation in community based programs or their own homes are provided through two therapeutic recreation programs (Vista Nueva East and West), the Live-In Registry, FSAL's Home Care Services (Homemakers/Home Health Aides), and the Personal Care housing units of Buena Vida. The four adult day-care programs (TELOCA, El Rinconcito, Sirrine, and Longview) complete the service network to those who do not require institutionalization. Buena Vida also provides beds for those who require nursing care.

The adult day-care services are enriched by cooperative arrangements with agencies such as Catholic Social Services of Phoenix and Tri-City CSS, the Visiting Nurse Service of Maricopa County, the Aging Division of the Human Resources Department of the City of Phoenix, City of Mesa, the Elderly Program of Phoenix South Mental Health Center, Tri-City Mental Health Center, the Easter Seal Society, and the American Red Cross. Each center also benefits from the availability of interdisciplinary graduate and undergraduate student teams from Arizona University's College of Nursing, School of Social Work, and Department of Recreation. Occupational therapy students have come to us from the University of Kansas and the University of Buffalo, and students in the Mental Health Technology Program of the Maricopa County Community College District have also participated in the adult day-care programs. A contract with the Arizona State Department of Economic Security for reimbursement of costs through Title XX funds provides the operating income for the three Level II day-care centers (TELOCA, El Rinconcito, and Sirrine). Longview Senior Center for Restorative Care (Level I) is funded by a Title III grant from the Area Agency on Aging (Region I—Maricopa County). Matching funds are currently provided by Maricopa County and the Mesa United Way. Private donations from innumerable sources and the ongoing support of groups such as Epsilon Sigma Alpha and the Sirrine Auxiliary provide scholarship funds for those who are not eligible for Title XX but cannot pay the net cost of care which, when two-way transportation is included, runs approximately $14 per day per person.

Despite the complexity and difficulty of funding the adult day-care services, our staff have managed to provide participants and their families with a unified program in which the participant/family is viewed as the client unit and in which continuity between program and home environment is promoted. Therapeutic intervention with the participant is facilitated by professional approaches to him within a context in which he is comfortable, primarily his activity program. Intervention with families begins within the educational context of evening "classes" that initially focus on helpful hints for easing the burden on families who care for elderly relatives.

Because staff do not insist upon the traditional therapeutic setting (private office or small group room), because staff are confident that they can function therapeutically without the customary props and structure, and because the day-care setting affords an opportunity for intensive and consistent intervention, frail older persons and their families experience positive personal and interpersonal growth. Many who viewed the adult day-care service as merely a temporary reprieve from institutional care have found it, instead, to be an exciting adventure, a gateway to personal growth and positive change.

4

The New Directions Workshop for Senior Citizens

Genevieve R. Meyer

Setting Up the Program

The idea of utilizing the Recreation and Parks Department as an avenue for reaching senior citizens in need of psychological assistance emerged in 1974, while I was conducting an informal interview study of well-adjusted seniors. I wanted to begin some kind of volunteer program, but first I needed to determine what kind of services to offer. The research literature was rich in material stressing loneliness, boredom, and isolation as important mental health problems of the 60-plus age group, but articles on solutions were sparse.

Stimulated by Maslow's (1954) method of looking for answers by studying the "well-adjusted" rather than the "maladjusted," I decided to identify a group of older adults who were leading meaningful and zestful lives and to ask them "how they were doing it." I enlisted the aid of the manager of the local Senior Citizens Center, which was under the Santa Monica Recreation and Parks Department, to help me find seniors living full and happy lives who would be willing to be interviewed.

This interview study led to the formulation of a New Directions Workshop Program, designed to help those older adults who were having difficulty with the transition into the freedom of the senior years and who needed to set new goals for themselves and to become solidly launched in movement toward those goals. In discussing with the Senior Citizens Center manager the logistics of how and where the workshop could best be held, she suggested using the Arts and Crafts Room in a park removed from the Senior Center itself. This had two advantages. First, any connotation of psychotherapy was avoided by offering the workshops through the Recreation and Parks Department. Second, any association with the prevailing "social club" image of the Senior Center was minimized by conducting the workshops in the separate park building which was, incidentally, easily reached by public transportation.

Regarding the logistics of cost and publicity, the Santa Monica Recreation and Parks Department was most helpful not only in providing the physical facilities, but also in sending out news releases and in announcing the workshop in its bulletin of activities, mailed to all Santa Monica residents four times a year. (An example is shown in Fig. 1.) As indicated earlier, the psychological services have been given on a volunteer basis; and beginning in Fall 1978, volunteer peer counselors have been added as co-leaders of the group.

The first workshop was offered in the summer of 1975. So far, fourteen workshops have been conducted, coordinated with the Fall, Winter, Spring, and Summer Programs of the Recreation and Parks Department. The size of the group is limited to fifteen, with an average of six to nine participants. Approximately 15 percent of them were male, the rest female. Participants have ranged in age from the mid-50s to mid-80s, with most in their 60s. The eight-session workshops meet weekly for one-and-a-half hours. They are free and open to anyone 50 years of age or older. Participants are welcome to re-enroll (and many of them do) if they need more than eight weeks to become secure with their new goals.

Carrying Out the Program

While the specific strategies and techniques have varied throughout the fourteen workshops, the basic objectives have proved to be both good and workable. The *first* objective is to develop a warm, trusting, and emotionally involving atmosphere in the group. The *second* objective is to develop awareness that new directions are available and to arouse the hope and confidence that it is possible for each person to establish new goals that will add richness to each person's daily life. The *third* objective consists of having each participant choose a definite goal on which he/she would like to work

Figure 1.

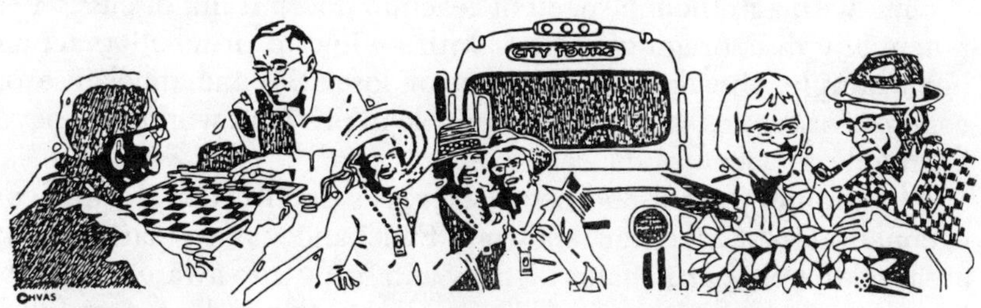

NEW DIRECTIONS WORKSHOP

WHEN: Fridays, October 6 - November 9
10:30 - 12 noon

WHERE: Lincoln Park Craft Room
1130 Lincoln Boulevard, Santa Monica

HOW TO REGISTER: Simply come to the first class session.
Anyone 50 years of age or over is welcome.
FREE!

WHAT IS IT? We will participate in informal discussions on new directions for the senior years, available community resources, experiences of moving toward new goals, self assertion, and clarification of values.

THE INSTRUCTOR IS: Dr. Genevive Meyer, School of Education, California State University, Los Angeles

Santa Monica Recreation and Parks Department
393-9975, EXT. 276

and then begin to take steps toward its realization. The group support and encouragement that emerges during this period sustains movement toward the individual goals and is invaluable in fostering genuine growth. The objectives are described in the opening session and are quietly maintained and reaffirmed throughout the later sessions, as needed.

In the first two sessions, the approach is "educational" in nature, with material presented by the leader/instructor designed to show the "positive" side of aging. This involves liberal mention of heartening research findings (for example, that intellectual capacities do not decline with age though speed of reaction does), frank discussion of potentially discouraging findings with a view to preventive action (for example, the theme of "use it or lose it"), and much use of concrete examples showing what people in previous workshops have been able to accomplish.

In addition, paper-and-pencil exercises (such as the Meyer Avocational Interest Inventory shown in Fig. 2 and Values Clarification) are used to help participants identify and bring into awareness existing areas in which they might like to develop themselves more fully, as well as new areas they might wish to explore. These are done in class/group time—usually one per group meeting. Afterward, the participants are asked to share with the group their two or three highest interest areas (from the Avocational Interest Inventory Profile) or several of the activities they really enjoy doing (from the Values Clarification Exercise).

Since the participants are seated around a table, it is quite natural to have each one speak in turn. This method has the advantage of allowing the leader, in an unobtrusive and subtle way, to intervene should any one member tend to monopolize the time, as well as to encourage any reticent member to share something about him/herself. It has been my observation that many people currently in their sixties or older have not had the opportunity to learn to function freely, easily, and on an "equal time" basis in a group milieu. This may be simply a generational or age-group difference that will cease to be relevant when those now in the younger age groups have reached their senior years, or it may apply to many people of all ages when they first come into a sharing-oriented group. In any case, it is necessary to allow time for group members to build the skills needed to function effectively in such a group setting. Using rather structured material in the first two sessions has the effect of permitting the participants to become accustomed to "appropriate ways of group interaction" before moving into the more unstructured sessions that follow.

The Case of Agatha

Take the case of Agatha as an example of growth in group communication skills. In the first session, her behavior toward the other group members was hostile and demanding. She seemed to want them to accord her "special and superior status" because of her brief career

Figure 2. Avocational Interest Inventory
by Genevieve R. Meyer, Ph.D.

Please rate each activity according to how much it appeals to you (even if you have not yet tried it), on a scale from 0 to 5. If you really like *it, write ":5" on the dotted line to the left of the statement. If you* dislike *it, write "0." If your feelings fall in between, write in the number (1, 2, 3, or 4) that feels best.*

RATING	ACTIVITIES	SCALE
....	Going to an art, sculpture, or crafts exhibit	
....	Reading about the lives or painting methods of artists	
....	Watching a TV program on the history of art and paintings of that period	A
	Circulating a petition or discussing politics	
....	Doing committee work on problems of senior citizens	
....	Attending a community meeting on environmental problems	B
....	Making models of ships, abstract forms, or dolls	
....	Sketching or painting (oils, water color, etc.)	
....	Designing and making pottery, collages, or leather work	C
....	Writing a short story, poem, or any other creative writing	
....	Reading a novel, play, poetry, or an autobiography	
....	Going to a play or little theatre performance	D
....	Playing any musical instrument or singing	
....	Listening to records or watching a musical show on TV	
....	Going to a concert, recital, or other musical production	E
....	Taking care of plants or visiting a botanical garden	
....	Watching birds or TV programs on nature or wildlife	
....	Watching the sunset; looking at the ocean, clouds, trees	F
....	Swimming, playing golf, or dancing	
....	Taking a stroll or a long walk	
....	Exercising (such as Yoga, Slim and Trim Classes, etc.)	G
....	Going to an exhibit at the Museum of Science & Industry	
....	Observing the stars or seeing a planetarium show	
....	Watching a science documentary on TV or reading about scientific subjects	H
....	Working or volunteering in a social service agency	
....	Doing things that make conditions better for others	
....	Helping your neighbors or friends when they have problems	I
....	Taking a local sight-seeing trip with a friendly group	
....	Watching a travelogue movie or TV show of foreign lands	
....	Touring a foreign country or taking a cruise	J

as a professional opera singer prior to her marriage. She frequently interrupted with questions that were directed to the group leader in a manner that tried to emotionally exclude the other participants and to shift the interaction into a one-to-one exchange with the instructor/leader. Apparently because this technique was discouraged by the leader's response that she should hold her questions/comments until it was her turn, she did not come to the second session. She did show up, however (late of course) for the third session, and immediately began the same kind of disruptive behavior of interrupting with questions or comments.

At this point, the leader introduced the concept of "creative listening." This involved the practice exercise of stopping the discussion every fifteen to twenty minutes and having each participant summarize what he/she thought the person who had been speaking had "really been saying." The participants were encouraged to attend to nonverbal cues, especially facial expressions, body language, and voice tone as they listened creatively to the words of the speaking participant.

These creative listening practice exercises were quite useful in quieting Agatha. By the fifth group meeting, the other participants were joining in the process of "taming Agatha" in a surprisingly friendly and jocular manner. For example, "Agatha, you're doing it again," said with a smile or laughter, became a common refrain from the other group members. By the end of the workshop, even Agatha was smiling and seemed fully at home in the group.

Such creative listening practice periods also serve to facilitate the growth of a genuinely involving and trusting group atmosphere. Meanwhile, the participants can carry on with the business of sharing and absorbing the high-interest areas and preferred activities indicated on the Avocational Interest Inventory and the Values Clarification Exercise worksheet filled out earlier by each participant.

As soon as the participants have some idea of their own high-interest areas, as well as those of the other group members, they are given the ongoing homework assignment of exploring the local community for announcements of any activities, course offerings, excursions, involvement opportunities, and the like that could relate to any high-interest area mentioned by any group member. At this stage, the role of the group leader shifts away from the educational/instructor function and toward that of group facilitator and resource person.

As the participants begin to share the results of their explorations, they become more involved, in the group and more aware of a larger world of opportunities available to them than their initial "tunnel vision" had allowed. The amount of laughter and good feeling that begins to emerge in the group life at this point really cannot be put into words.

The Case of Mabel and Louis

Mabel and Louis became avid explorers of the free programs and "goodies" offered by the many banks in the area that were promoting their services for senior citizens. At this time, the other participants in that particular workshop were bringing in every week the more usual, and very helpful, information about such activities as one-day or weekend group excursions sponsored by senior citizen centers, lectures and book review meetings given at the libraries, academic and recreational courses available at the Emeritus College (a division of the local community college specifically geared to the interests of seniors), free art exhibits and concerts, and announcements of "involvement opportunities" from the newspapers and TV public service ads. Meanwhile, Mabel and Louis kept turning up new banks to visit. Every week they would arrive with free movie tickets from one or another of the banks.

This organized search for banks stemmed partly from Louis's need for a structured schedule. He had just retired, and expressed bitter feelings about the impersonal handling of his retirement luncheon—especially after so many years of service to the same company. He was approaching his retirement like "work," and every night he and Mabel would draw up a schedule for the following day.

Their goal of exploring the community for available resources led them not only to banks, but also to walking tours, visiting the art and science museums, and attending the film series offered free at the local library. Both seemed to be enjoying a revitalized relationship as a couple.

By the third group session, Louis was no longer the bitter man who had leaned forward, angry and tense, eager to berate his former employer. Instead, he was smiling and sat back in his chair in a more assured posture. Being the only male in that workshop also helped to foster the regrowth of his self-esteem. By the seventh group meeting, his walk was jaunty and his demeanor enthusiastic as he and Mabel entered the group session room, eager to relate their latest "bank find."

At that point, Louis's company asked him to return as a part-time consultant; that really seemed to clear away any residual feelings of "having been pushed out." He said he would need to drop out of the group, though Mabel would continue. During the eighth session, while the group was expressing feelings of missing Louis, in he walked. He explained that, as consultant, he felt he could just tell the company he was taking two hours off. He had been sitting at his desk, missing the group, and realized not only that he would prefer being at the group meeting but that he had the freedom to schedule his life the way he wished.

In Louis's case, he had found the new direction that was right for him. It was not a new hobby or job that he needed, but rather a different approach to living, characterized by an openness to new experiences he could add to the existing structure of his daily life. Such new experiences included a cross-country trip the couple took after the workshop, organized around visiting relatives plus Boston and Washington, D.C., which they had never seen. These experiences more than compensated for the eight-to-five work routine from which Louis had retired. In his case, the transition into the senior years was made with relative ease and the prognosis for a more rewarding life as a couple appeared to be excellent.

For some people, the transition is not marked by abrupt and/or obvious turning points (such as retirement or the death of a spouse). It is more subtle and gradual, rather like a continually shifting adaptation process to the various changes that do occur in the "outer" conditions of a person's life.

In Mabel's case, the change in her outer conditions was her husband's retirement. While she was in the group, her new directions emerged gently as, willingly and eagerly she went along with Louis's explorations. Indeed, she reaped her own benefits from his organized explorations and appeared to be pleasantly surprised by the enlarging of her sphere of activities. The only issues that she brought out on her own concerned the changing relationship with her daughter-in-law, who was nearing the birth of her second child. Some friction was developing due to Mabel's strong need to involve herself in getting things set up for the baby's arrival. Discussion of this problem at several group meetings facilitated a more relaxed, "hands-off" attitude on Mabel's part. Of course, the diverting of much of her time and energy into her explorations with Louis was a large factor in her growth toward a more comfortable relationship with her daughter-in-law.

Treating Human Relations Problems

The whole area of difficulties in human relationships (whether due to problems with others, such as family and/or neighbors, or due to loneliness resulting from a lack of significant others in one's life) seemed to me to be a basic issue in all fourteen of the workshops. Typically these problems were rarely announced "up front." Sometimes they came up, almost as "an aside," when the participant was working on a more socially acceptable growth goal (e.g., how to adjust to other people in emeritus college classes that the participant was taking to explore the *goal* of further education). At other times, discussion of interpersonal problems was stimulated when the group leader would deliberately introduced that topic (usually in relation to presenting material on assertion training with accompanying practice exercises).

Case Examples

Josephine. Josephine was a widow approaching 60 who lived alone and augmented her private fixed income with part-time salesclerk jobs. After reviewing her high interest scores in "Literary and Musical Activities" and in "Trips and Travel" on the Avocational Interest Inventory, she came up with the idea of taking a trip to Hawaii and asked the group for advice on the merit of her plan. The ensuing discussion uncovered the real cause of Josephine's uncertainty. She was caught between the desire to spend her limited resources for her own needs and the feeling that she "ought to" help out her married daughter with her money problems. Naturally this led to considerable group discussion on relationships and responsibilities between parents and children from which the whole group benefited. As for Josephine, not only did she free herself from an excessive sense of responsibility toward her daughter, but also she discovered that travel per se was not of genuine importance to her. Instead she got involved in drama classes at the community college. Acting had been a longstanding interest of hers, and she began to create her own "one-woman comedy skits." After trying them out both in class and in the group, she began to perform at church social affairs. I have met Josephine on several occasions over the past three years, and she is still writing and performing her own material.

Edith. The lack of satisfying human contact is illustrated in the case of Edith. She had been retired for several years from her job as a social worker. On the surface, she seemed to be a "very together lady" whose only problem was too much time on her hands. She began exploring political activity as her goal by attending both League of Women Voters' and Gray Panthers' meetings.

In the course of sharing her reactions to those groups with the Workshop participants, she casually mentioned that she found the apartment building in which she lived to be an unfriendly place and that she would prefer more day-to-day interchange with her neighbors. During the next meeting at which her "situation" was discussed, she came to the realization that what she really missed was the kind of interaction she had shared with her "office family" before she retired. This did not come out until the last workshop session, so Edith was one of those who enrolled in a second workshop.

During her second series of group sessions, she switched her goal to exploring alternative living arrangements. Before the end of her second workshop, Edith had purchased a condominium in a development for seniors near Santa Barbara. Before buying, she had spent a weekend there visiting a friend she had previously made through work. Upon experiencing the kind of community feeling in that development, she quickly decided it was the right place for her. She came back to visit the group after she had moved and she seemed very content with her choice.

Moving Beyond the Work Ethic

Another basic issue that has emerged in all of the workshops is the need to move beyond the "work ethic" values of the middle years and to develop new yardsticks for measuring "what makes life worth living." Perseverence, industriousness, competence, and achievement are splendid values; but expression of the growth needs (also called "being values" and "meta-needs") that Maslow (1968) includes in self-actualization requires the development of other virtues as well. The cultivation of "aliveness, individuality, playfulness, effortlessness, goodness, and meaningfulness" (and these represent less than half of Maslow's list) seems especially appropriate during the senior years. While it would be ideal for all of us to be self-actualizing all of the time, that is not the case. However, the freedom and leisure of the senior years can provide the conditions for more self-actualizing to occur.

The two major barriers to such growth that I have observed in the workshops have been difficulty in relating to others and lack of a rich development of values due to overemphasis on "work-related values." Typically these problems surface both in the *awareness phase* (when participants are exploring possible new directions and coming to realize that they can set new goals for themselves) and in the *commitment and follow-through phase* (when participants are choosing goals and taking steps to fulfill them).

To return to the case of Edith, she had made real progress in seeing that a need for more satisfying social relationships was part of her problem and in taking steps to change her living arrangements. Yet her loyalty to her "work-ethic values" remained as the other major barrier to a meaningful and psychologically nourishing use of her leisure time.

During her many working years in the social service field, she had grown accustomed to viewing her role in the world through glasses whose lenses were colored by duty and responsibility and to measuring her self-worth by the yardstick of how much she was able to help those in need of social work services. She only too naturally carried those values over into her initial choice of possible new directions for leisure time activities (namely, volunteer political action with either the League of Women Voters or the Gray Panthers).

It took several group sessions in which values clarification and brainstorming exercises were done and disucssed before Edith began to get in touch with her dormant needs for other kinds of life experiences. In opening up the topic "What does being productive mean to each one of you?," the group leader encouraged the group to think out loud in an almost free associative manner as to what kinds of things really made them feel useful throughout the course of their daily activities. Afterwards, the participants discussed to what extent their individual feelings of usefulness/productivity were determined by their own inner choices, and to what extent they were influenced by standards they had uncritically absorbed from outside sources (e.g., parents, teachers, community leaders, books, and even commercial advertising).

In Edith's case, she began to reassess what values were truly important to her, which ones she would like to outgrow or discard, and what new ones she might like to develop. During this period her behavior in the group became lighter and freer and her general attitude seemed less serious and more playful. She quickly dropped her talk of volunteer political activity and went instead on some local, one-day group excursion tours to broaden her search for alternative living arrangements. It wasn't long before she began to consider the possibilities of foreign travel via group tours.

When Edith came back to visit the group after having moved to her new condominium, she was planning to take a group tour abroad and her enthusiasm bespoke a genuine inner excitement rather than a superficial attempt to fill up her free time. While I have not heard from Edith since that group session, my guess is that she will eventually include some political activity in her life. My guess is based on my observations of other participants who, after a period of euphoric absorption with the new horizons opened up by extending their values beyond those related to the "work ethic," gradually settle into a re-balanced pattern of life that includes both the new values and all of the old ones that are personally authentic.

Learning to Use Leisure Time

The whole area of leisure time planning can become very muddled indeed, especially when the old nostrums of "retirement is the time to relax and enjoy life" and "now is the time to take the trip you have always dreamed of" are applied. People who have never spent long periods away from home or have not developed inwardly satisfying hobbies prior to their 60s usually have a difficult time when they first try to "enjoy their leisure." The first step in helping such workshop participants is simply to explain to them that it takes learning and practice to acquire the skills necessary *to travel* easily and pleasurably or *to play* authentically so that the hobby/activity is genuinely satisfying rather than a time-filler/killer.

The knowledge that they are not abnormal can bring immediate relief. The second step, which is more difficult, is to help them understand that the learning process with respect to leisure-time activities requires a somewhat different attitude from the one that they used when learning school material or work skills. This difference can best be described as "letting it happen" (with respect to play) versus "making it happen" (with respect to work). The third step involves thoughtful selection of the new directions to be explored; and this step is greatly facilitated by additional values clarification exercises plus the ongoing sharing of each participant's exploration of community resources.

The last step depends primarily on the group members themselves. The encouragement and acceptance they give one another is invaluable in enabling participants to persevere in moving toward their individual goals.

Case Example

Pauline. Pauline had just retired from a rigorously scheduled job as a court reporter when she enrolled in her first workshop. She was apprehensive about money and uncertain as to how it would work out to have so much time at home with her husband. He had retired several years earlier and had urged her to retire so they could have more time together. According to Pauline, her husband was quite relaxed and comfortable in his adjustment to a retired life-style. Underneath, she rather disapproved of his easy-going attitude and expressed concern that she might become as "disorganized and casual" as he seemed to be to her as she looked at him through her work-ethic glasses colored "efficiency" and "get it done on time." In the second group meeting, she said she was thinking of getting a part-time job to finance a trip to Hawaii. At this point the group leader suggested she postpone any decisions until she saw the results of the group's exploration of community resources. By the fourth session, she was beginning to experience the effect of the values clarification exercises and to tone down her need for immediate action.

As Pauline settled into a more patient consideration of the options available, she became intrigued with the varied offerings of the Emeritus College (associated with the local community college) and decided to register for some classes as *her new direction.* However, her ingrained work ethic values began to intrude again when she started making her curriculum selections. For example, the acting class had really caught her fancy; but she felt she ought to take something more educational (like philosophy) instead. Also, she was torn between her still-present need to schedule her time efficiently and the fact that there was a conflict in the times that the courses she thought she wanted were offered. Group discussion of this problem also turned up a deep fear on her part that she might not excel at her studies (having never gone beyond high school academic subjects) or that she might find herself committed to a class that might turn out to be either too hard or too boring.

The continued gentle support and jovial reinforcement that Pauline received from the other participants during this phase of her growth was invaluable. She gradually came to see that she had the right to drop courses if she did not like them and to allocate her study time according to how much each course meant to her. She did take the acting class and enjoyed it thoroughly, spending most of her time and energy there while doing adequate, though less, work in her other classes. In fact Pauline's growth into her new attitude toward learning facilitated change in the way other participants approached their new activities. There was more freedom in trying things on for size, with just enough perseverance to see if the activity or hobby was really worth pursuing; and there was less emphasis on outer yardsticks (e.g., the opinions of others or how well or fast they learned and produced in comparison to others). In short, they were discovering their own inner yardsticks.

Pauline was one of those who both needed and wanted to sign up for a second workshop before she could feel solidly launched in her new directions. By that time her fascination with the Emeritus College classes was beginning to wane and she was putting her life in balance on a broader and more self-actualizing basis. She did take a part-time job since she discovered she truly did want some paid work activity in her life. She started taking tennis lessons with her husband and appeared to be calmly building toward a richer relationship with him. At that point she decided to explore her social service interests (which had been high on the Avocational Interest Inventory). Unlike Edith, her work years had been spent in technical work with little deep human contact. So it was appropriate for her to want to reach out toward helping others, even as it had been appropriate for Edith to grow beyond her exclusive devotion to serving the needs of others.

As Pauline was looking into the RSVP programs, she came across the Information Booth on the town's main shopping mall. She discovered that volunteers worked there, answering both visitors' and sightseers' questions as well as referring senior citizens to appropriate agencies. While discussing this in the workshop, she was able to voice her feelings of inadequacy. She knew she had been a good court reporter, but she doubted whether she had any talent for working in a service capacity with people and worried about her lack of experience and knowledge in that field. Through the encouragement of the group, she found the courage to make inquiries and was very quickly signed up to volunteer at the mall booth. Shortly after starting her assignment there, the workshop ended.

I have seen Pauline on many occasions since then over the past four years, as we live in the same neighborhood. It has been both rewarding and refreshing to see the self-actualization process unfold once it has been stimulated by programs such as the New Directions Workshop.

After several months of service in the booth on the mall, Pauline had gained considerable self-confidence. (Incidentally, I heard from her supervisor that the organizational skills she had developed during her working career had been instrumental in making her one of their most effective volunteers.) She felt she had outgrown the mall booth, since it was limited to rather brief contacts with people while their questions were being answered. On her own, she began to inquire about other service opportunities. Through friends at her church, she heard about the Meals-on-Wheels Program; and she and her husband have jointly worked one day a week delivering meals for at least the last two years. They have both found the continuing weekly contact with the same people to be extremely gratifying.

One thing has led to another, and at present this friendly, enthusiastic couple have enlarged their service sphere to include monthly outings with a group of mentally retarded teenage girls who have adopted them as their "unoffical grandparents." They also have established a regular weekly routine of visiting several nursing homes in the area. One powerful image I think I shall always remember is of Pauline's husband's buoyant and cheerful face when he said, in a recent conversation, that they were busier and happier in their retirement years than either of them had ever been during their working careers.

Naturally it is impossible to tell what their lives would be like now without the early intervention of the New Directions Workshop. Pauline told me several years after that she had been so full of anxiety that she was a "basket case" when she enrolled in her first workshop; and she at least is convinced that her experiences in those two workshops were instrumental in shaping her present life. Whether or not that is a realistic assessment, it is probably true that Pauline would not have sought help through the traditional psychotherapeutic avenues during that troubled transition period in her life.

Levels in the Counseling Process

In Pauline's case several levels of the counseling/psychotherapy process can be seen at work, in addition to the "working through" of her anxiety referred to above. At one level there was the probable *prevention* of friction and possible deterioration in her relationship with her husband by early intervention. At another level, there was the *supportive maintenance* of adequate social relationships through her weekly interaction with other workshop participants. At yet other levels, both *avocational counseling* and *self-actualization* came into play.

Thus, the flexible format of the New Directions Workshop Program can accommodate various kinds of psychological growth and can attract people in need of psychological services who might otherwise be put off by the labels of "counseling" or "psychotherapy." Of course it is not designed to handle deep problems, and any such cases should be referred elsewhere.

Case Example

Vivian. Vivian had recently retired after many years in civil service (with primarily clerical responsibilities) and had just moved to California from New York. On the surface, her problem appeared to be that of finding new social relationships and making the adjustment to living in an entirely different kind of climate and community. After a later session when she seemed to be quite discouraged with her lack of progress in adapting to southern California living, I felt quite concerned about her obvious depression and invited her to have coffee with me. The ensuing discussion revealed that her sister, with whom she had planned to retire to Florida, had committed suicide just prior to their moving date.

After that, Vivian could not bear the thought of the Florida move and hastily came to California instead. Since I was already familiar with Vivian's strong involvement with her church in New York and her inability to locate one in this area in which she could feel comfortable, I offered to find out about pastoral counselors for her. Luckily, I was able to find an excellent one in her neighborhood who belonged to the same denomination.

Vivian did go for counseling with him, and it turned out to be quite helpful. In a letter she wrote me some months later, she said she had come to terms with her sister's death. Also she had again become very involved in church activities and had made several new friends; she was now feeling very content with her move to California.

A Summary of the Psychological Methods Adapted for Use in the Program

Throughout the course of the fourteen workshops completed to date, various psychological approaches and techniques have been tried. This section is a summary of those that have proved most helpful with the older adults that have participated in the workshops.

Stress Is Learned—But So Is Relaxation!

In 1977 Dr. Meyer started a Stress Reduction Clinic for the Santa Monica Bay Area Health Screening Clinic for the Elderly. Originally a biweekly drop-in clinic for patients with high blood pressure problems, it has evolved into a twelve-week program designed to help the over-60 group to cope with stress. The sessions cover relaxation, deep breathing, progressive muscular relaxation, guided imagery, autoregulation, and stress management.

After becoming acquainted with Hans Selye on stress and Herbert Benson on the relaxation response, the twelve individuals first practice relaxation in the group. Later they discuss their daily home practice of the techniques learned, ironing out any problems encountered and adding variations on the basic relaxation response. The other techniques are demonstrated and practiced in the sessions that follow. The holistic approach is emphasized, and participants are encouraged to develop their own methods of utilizing the basic techniques. If they wish they can continue in an advanced group.

Gladys exemplifies the results that can be achieved with persistent daily practice. She was referred to the Stress Reduction Clinic for hypertension. Her physician had tried several types of medication, but the side effects made Gladys sick. Retirement from her job did reduce the original reading of 210/110, but a return to part-time volunteer work sent it up again to 198/98. Neither improved diet nor increased rest brought the figure down, so she was highly motivated when she began the program.

Gladys describes herself as having always been a tense, jumpy person. She says that the breathing techniques produced the first noticeable effects, in that she slept better and no longer had headaches. Other effects were psychological; using the relaxation response changed her whole life-style. She always practices it morning and night, and usually in the afternoon at the convalescent hospital where she works part-time as a volunteer. If she skips the afternoon practice she reports an immediate rise in her irritability level and her sensitivity to pressure.

After one month, Gladys had her first blood pressure check and was told it had started to come down; the trend has continued until at the end of three months the reading was 178/90. She expects to reduce it still further in the advanced group. Meanwhile she feels much happier; as she puts it, "even my driving is calmer and slower."

Transactional Analysis has been a good source for concepts. I have modified the "I'm OK, You're OK" position to "I'm Important, You're Important" (following the suggestion of a colleague who has been using TA for some time with seniors). The "I'm OK" statement can be easily misinterpreted as referring to physical health. After explaining in the first group meeting that a trusting and cooperative atmosphere is necessary for working effectively as a group, the "I'm Important, You're Important" position is introduced, plus the concept of positive and negative "strokes." These then become the basic ground rules for group interaction, and participants are encouraged to give positive feedback to each other as soon as they begin sharing the results of their exploration of community resources.

Negative feedback is discouraged on the basis that there is already enough of it available for seniors in their daily lives. This in itself can stimulate lively discussion of the many negative attitudes toward aging and older people that the participants have encountered in our youth-oriented society. If the discussion becomes too long and drawn out to be productive, the "ain't it awful" game is briefly described and then discouraged on the basis that it is not conducive to selecting and working toward viable new directions.

Assertion Training techniques have been very useful and are usually introduced when the group reaches the stage of working on goals related to building and/or improving social relationships. Of the various assertion training exercises, the one that has been most frequently used is self-disclosure (see Smith, 1975). Participants enjoy practicing this exercise as a method for getting conversation started when their goal is to make new friends (e.g., in Emeritus College classes).

Values clarification exercises have consistently proved very helpful and have been used in every workshop. Of the many publications out on that topic, the paperback entitled *Values Clarification* (Simon, Howe, and Kirschenbaum, 1972) has a number of exercises that can easily be adapted for use with senior citizens. The first one listed, called "Twenty Things You Love to Do," has regularly been employed, along with any others that seem appropriate to the particular goals on which the various participants are working.

The technique of brainstorming, once it is described as having its widest use in the business world, is easily accepted and learned by seniors. It can be adapted to fit any topic and has the special advantage of enabling the participants to go below their surface thinking and get in touch with their deeper feelings and attitudes. It has also been useful in generating unique and creative ways of approaching any unusual new direction that a participant may come up with.

As for the underlying theoretical approach of the group leader, a combination of Erikson's description of the eight stages of man's psychological development with Maslow's description of the self-actualization process plus his theory of needs (especially the growth needs) has proved very fruitful indeed (Erikson, 1963, Chap. 7; Maslow, 1968). Since the New Directions Workshop is definitely not a course in psychological theories, the works of Erikson and Maslow are not gone into in depth, though references are freely given when requested. Participants also receive a list of popular books on aging available at the local public library. They are encouraged to do as much outside reading as they wish, since the more effort they put into the workshop, the more they get out of it.

It is my personal belief that Erikson's view of the mature or senior years (the eighth stage) is valid in its delineation of the growth challenge unique to those years as the development of "ego integrity" (vs. despair). The basic purpose of the New Directions Workshop Program is to prevent a descent into despair and to facilitate the emergence of ego integrity, as described in the case examples presented throughout this chapter.

Recommended Readings

Alberti, R., and Emmons, M. *Your perfect right—a guide to assertive behavior.* San Luis Obispo, CA: Impace, 1970.

Benson, H. *The relaxation response.* New York: Avon, 1975.

Cabot, N. H. *You can't count on dying.* New York: Houghton, Mifflin, 1961.

Comfort, A. *A good age.* New York: Simon and Schuster, 1976.

DeBeauvoir, S. *The coming of age.* New York: Putnam, 1972.

Erikson, E. H. *Childhood and society.* New York: Norton, 2nd ed., 1963.

Goble, F. *The third force: the psychology of Abraham Maslow.* New York: Pocket Books, 1971.

Harris, T. A. *I'm OK—you're OK.* New York: Avon Books, 1967.

Hart, M. *When your husband retires.* New York: Appleton-Century-Crofts, 1960.

Kanin, G. *It takes a long time to become young.* New York: Doubleday, 1978.

Selye, H. *Stress without distress.* New York: Signet, 1974.

Simon, S. B., Howe, L. W. and Kirschenbaum, H. *Values clarification.* New York: Hart, 1972.

5

Therapy Approaches with Rural Elders

Russell A. Dunckley, Candida J. Lutes, Judith N. Wooten, and Robert A. Kooken

Providing psychological services to rural elders is an area that has been largely overlooked. Although about 40 percent of older people live in nonmetropolitan areas (35 percent in small towns and 5 percent on farms; Butler and Lewis, 1977), virtually all of the work that has been reported by mental health practitioners has been accumulated from work with elders in cities, and the majority of services are designed to be delivered in metropolitan areas. In this chapter we are concerned with the delivery of psychological services to aged populations in rural areas. By "psychological services" we mean those involving the aged client's personal cares, concerns, and worries, regardless of whether these are addressed by a psychologist, social worker, minister, physician, friend, or member of the family.

The present chapter is an initial attempt to deal with the special problems that arise in rural areas. In considering these problems, one must remember that the needs are much the same in rural areas as in urban settings, but that the resources, service attitudes, and philosophies are likely to differ in many ways. Regardless of age, social class, or place of residence, all people need to have satisfactory health, good nutrition, recreation, a sense of safety, privacy, a sense of purpose or productivity, a sense of being able to cope with problems, a sense of being needed and appreciated by others, and someone to go to in a crisis. The fewer of these that are present, the more likely that the person will be unhappy, lonely, and unable to cope.

Limitations and Resources in Rural Areas

Problems in Service Delivery in Rural Settings

Even though the needs in rural areas are very similar to those in urban areas, the rural aged present some special problems in terms of delivering psychological services. It is important to outline some of those problems here because any therapy approach, whether traditional or nontraditional, must deal with them in one way or another.

First of all, rural elders have fewer resources to work with in many areas than do their urban counterparts. For example, the rural aged are poorer; according to the 1970 Census (Noll, 1978), 81 percent of rural elders had annual incomes below $4,000, and fully 61 percent had annual incomes below $2,000. In terms of housing, rural elders were more likely to own their own homes than urban elders (82 percent of rural elders own their own homes), yet 60 percent of rural elders lived in a home that was at least 40 years old, the median value of these homes was $8,000, and more than 20 percent of these homes lacked complete plumbing. According to articles reviewed by Lawton (1977), rural elders are more likely to be in poorer health than their urban counterparts and to receive less frequent medical care, and according to unpublished data that we have collected on over 1,100 aged Texans, rural elders have somewhat less confidence in their doctors and are somewhat less likely to think that the physicians' primary interest is in their health rather than their money.

A second problem in delivering services to rural elders is one of communication. Research has demonstrated that rural elders are less likely to be aware of social services that are available (as reviewed by Lawton, 1977), and it has been our experience that even when they are aware of the existence of a social service agency, they may not be aware that it provides services that they might consider appropriate for themselves. For example, in our work with a rural mental health outreach clinic we have found that aged clients (as well as others) assume that the only function of the clinic is to assist in commitments to the state hospital and after-care for people who are "crazy." They are often completely unaware of the range of services available to "normal" individuals, as well as of the fact that the vast majority of our clients are normal. It is important to note at this point that we have encountered the same beliefs among service providers in the area, such as ministers, physicians, and law enforcement officials.

If they are aware that such services exist, a third problem in delivering psychological services in rural areas involves their attitudes and beliefs about accepting assistance with psychological problems. Due to their financial situation, very few of the aged are in a position to pay for services, yet these clients have a strong need to perceive services as having been earned (Moen, 1978). Therefore, even if psychological services are thought to be needed, they may not be seen as accessible through traditional channels, such as agencies or private practitioners. In addition, we have found after becoming acquainted with clients that a major barrier they overcame within themselves before seeking assistance was the concept that one should be able to handle one's own problems and not need to rely on others.

There is also a problem in small communities in that it is very difficult to seek out psychological services anonymously. Aged clients are generally well-known in a small community, and they find it embarrassing to be seen going into a mental health clinic, sitting in the waiting room, or having their car parked outside. We have found this problem can be alleviated somewhat if the mental health clinic is located in the same building as other more acceptable services.

A fourth problem in delivering services to rural elders is transportation. For example, according to the 1970 Census, only 30 percent of rural elders have an automobile available (Noll, 1978), and rural areas generally lack any sort of public transportation. The roads are often in poor repair, there are longer distances between each person's home and available resources, many older people cannot afford to maintain their own cars, and many older people have suffered losses in vision or hearing that make it unsafe for them to drive. It has not been at all unusual for us to find that aged clients have had to pay a neighbor or family member for transportation. Some rural areas have transportation available to elders, but it is often available only for certain services and frequently is unreliable. For example, those clients who are willing to come to an outreach mental health clinic often must arrive hours before their appointment to be able to use the transportation, or often the transportation arrives too late for them to keep the appointment they have scheduled. In addition, the transportation is often not well-designed to accommodate the needs of the handicapped.

A fifth problem in delivering services in rural areas has to do with funding. The low population density in rural areas makes services much more expensive to deliver. In addition, obtaining local funds to serve as a match for federal funds for programs is extremely difficult, and the ability to finance services on a long-term basis is very low (Berry, 1978).

Thus, there are definite problems involved in delivering services to rural elders, and it is, of course, important to be aware of the barriers that may be encountered in such an enterprise. However, it is our contention that perhaps too much attention has been focused on identifying the barriers involved in delivering services in rural areas and not enough attention has been focused on the assets and resources available in these areas. If psychological services are to be made available to rural elders, then perhaps the available resources are a more important focus than the limitations.

Resources in Rural Settings

A major resource for rural elders is the support group made up of their friends and family. Rural elders have generally lived in their community for much longer than urban elders, and because of this length of residence and the size of the community the rural elder has more extensive relationships with others in his/her community. Unpublished data that we have gathered indicate that rural elders have the same amount of contact with their children and grandchildren as urban elders, although some authors have reported they may have slightly less contact (Bultena, 1969; Lawton, 1977). However, both in data we have collected and in that from other investigators (Bultena, 1969; Lawton, 1977), rural elders have more contact with their friends and more contact with their brothers and sisters. In addition, data we have collected indicate that rural elders who receive social services report that they receive more frequent visits from their social workers than do urban recipients. We have also collected data on the extent to which elders in rural and urban areas feel that they have someone they can confide in regarding such personal issues as concerns about their health, about death and dying, and about making plans for the future. We have found that the majority of elders report having someone they can confide in, and that there were no differences between rural and urban elders on this dimension.

An additional resource, in our view, lies in the fact that although rural elders have fewer resources available and less access to those that are available, they are less reticent than their urban counterparts to express the need for access to resources (Lawton, 1977). In addition, according to data we have gathered, the rural aged express more interest in visiting others and being visited by others than do the urban aged. Also, rural males who do not have someone in whom they can confide are more likely than urban males to indicate they would like to have someone to fill this function for them.

We have also found an additional resource among those who provide services in rural areas, where there is, of course, a much more restricted range of services available. It has been our experience that those who provide services in rural areas have a fairly broad concept of their jobs, so that they are quite willing to help the aged with problems they have identified even when they fall outside of the scope of their traditional job definition.

Younger elders as well as those who are not aged are more likely to see services as being acceptable than are older elders. This serves as a resource in two respects. In one respect it suggests that services are becoming more acceptable and the barriers against service use are being lowered somewhat. In a second respect, this suggests that since younger people are more willing to seek out services, they can be used as a resource in providing services to older friends and members of their families.

Providing Psychological Services to Rural Elders

Most of the work we have done in providing psychological services to rural elders has been through a rural outreach mental health clinic which also serves as a training site for some of our graduate students in psychology who are interested in rural mental health. Many of the workshops and groups for elders have been conducted through the University's Department of Psychology, although they would be just as feasible through the outreach clinic. The work through the outreach clinic is funded by the State's mental health system, which pays consultant fees to professional staff and provides travel reimbursements to the graduate students.

Our approach in providing psychological services to rural elders has generally proceeded along two different lines. The first of these has been to make traditional therapeutic services more acceptable, and the second has been to use nontraditional avenues to provide therapy to the aged and their families. We will attempt to show as we discuss each of these areas how we have tried to minimize the barriers to therapy among the aged and capitalize on the available resources.

Making Traditional Services More Acceptable

It is our feeling that programs with the aged should include as one aspect efforts to make traditional therapy approaches more acceptable. Every therapeutic modality has advantages and disadvantages, and there are some problems that are most adequately addressed by having an individual, couple, or family engage in traditional therapy with one or more therapists. We have attempted to approach this problem in essentially two ways.

Community education. Our first approach to making traditional services more acceptable is not really a separate effort but has been incorporated into our other efforts described below. In general this has consisted of reeducating the community. This has been attempted both through our meetings with other service providers and through workshops, meetings with church and civic groups, and so forth. We have continually found in doing this in rural areas that apart from the stigma attached to psychological services, many people are genuinely surprised to learn that psychologists work with people who aren't disturbed or "crazy" and that the kinds of services available include assisting normal people with the stresses of everyday life.

Interactions with other service providers. Our second approach to making traditional services more acceptable has been directed toward other service providers in the community, by whom we mean social workers, nurses, attorneys, ministers, police officers, and any other member of the community who is likely to be interacting with aged clients or their families at a point of crisis. Our work with them has generally involved four steps.

The first step hinges on the fact that in rural areas, the importance of developing personal relationships is critical. We have found that psychologists and others who provide social services are regarded with a certain amount of mistrust in rural areas and that professional qualifications in this area are met with a mixture of envy and mistrust that can easily turn into a lack of cooperation. Overcoming these attitudes with a friendly, accepting, and noncondescending attitude is a prerequisite to being considered a legitimate source of aid in the community.

Our second step in working with other service providers has been to communicate clearly and concretely what kinds of services are available. We begin by trying actively and directly to dispel myths that surround psychological services. For example, in telling other service providers that we work mostly with "normal" individuals and families, we have typically found that other service providers are quite surprised to learn that those kinds of services are available. They too have always thought that psychologists deal only with people who are "crazy." In addition, we provide concrete examples of the kinds of difficulties that we deal with. We might tell a police officer, for example, that we can assist with problems that arise between aging parents and their children, or in assisting a widow adjust to the loss of her spouse. This is, of course, accomplished without reference to a specific person in the community in order to maintain confidentiality. Since they are generally unfamiliar with what is involved in psychological services, the more concrete examples provided, the better.

Our third step in working with other service providers is to attempt to point out to them how the services we provide can alleviate some of the pressures they encounter in their own work. For example, police officers are frequently called upon to intervene in family disputes, and particularly in rural areas they may feel they do not have the tools available for dealing with these situations. In this case, psychological services can fill a gap in services of which the police officer is only too well aware. We have found it important in doing this to point out to other service providers what are appropriate and inappropriate referrals. For example, we point out to police officers that in order for us to be effective, people must come to us voluntarily and be motivated to produce changes.

The fourth step in working with other service providers is to do the things necessary to maintain the relationship over time and to establish and maintain credibility. This means, first of all, that when we communicate with service providers, we give them a realistic picture of what is possible. It also means maintaining clear and frequent communications. We have found, for example, that initial referrals to the clinic are often inappropriate. Maintaining a working relationship with the referral source requires patient, nonthreatening, and clear communications on making appropriate referrals.

It is important to point out at this juncture that we have found these steps to be more effective if we establish and maintain contacts with the other service providers in rural areas who are involved in actual service delivery. For example, we have found discussions with county judges and county sheriffs to be relatively fruitless in terms of generating referrals to the clinic since these positions in rural counties are largely administrative (although the importance of maintaining good relationships with these officials in a rural county cannot be overemphasized). However, discussion with police officers, county attorneys, ministers, and others who come into face-to-face contact with community problems has been more effective. We have found that direct service deliverers are very aware of the problems that might be appropriate for referral to the clinic. We have continually been impressed by the understanding, sensitivity, and concern they have for the people they work with.

The reception we have had in meetings with other service providers has varied greatly. For the most part we were pleased to find that we were given a warm reception which resulted in subsequent referrals to the clinic. Further, quite often the service provider we spoke with came to the clinic later with a concern about himself or a member of his family. However, we also encountered those who gave us a polite, although indifferent, hearing, and from whom we never heard again. We have also encountered other service providers who have discouraged people from coming to the clinic. For instance, whenever one local minister discovers that one of his parishioners is coming to the clinic, he approaches the parishioner and berates him for not coming to him first. Some clients are able to withstand this pressure and continue to come to the clinic, while others drop out as a result.

Nontraditional Approaches to Delivering Psychological Services

We have also explored a variety of nontraditional approaches to doing therapy with the aged, which are directed toward both other service providers and the aged and their families. These approaches have included reciprocal consultation with other service providers, workshops that are directed toward both other service providers and the aged and their families, and nontraditional groups with the aged.

Reciprocal consultation with other service providers. Given the importance of informal communication networks in rural areas, we have made efforts to meet with ministers, social workers, rehabilitation counselors, and other service providers in the area to exchange information and to make our respective resources accessible to each other. As we do this, we have essentially two goals in mind for these meetings.

Our first goal involves the fact that ministers, social workers, etc., in the community engage in a lot of work that is essentially therapy. Ministers in particular are often seen as a more legitimate source of assistance for personal concerns than are other service providers in rural areas. However, the amount of training and expertise that these other service providers have varies greatly, and our first goal is to put our background and experience at their disposal in assisting them in being more effective in what they do. Therefore, when we inform them of the services we offer, we also offer to consult with them on any cases in which they would like to call on us. We have again found that this offer is met in a variety of ways. Some service providers now call us on a frequent and regular basis with the problems they encounter, while others give us a polite hearing and are never heard from again.

Our second goal is to gain access to the resources available through these other service providers. For example, in rural communities the church may be the major focus of social activity outside the home. In addition to religious activities and social groups, many churches have initiated phone visitation programs whereby church members who are unable to get out of their homes may continue to feel they are fulfilling useful functions by calling others who are ill or shut-in. Therefore, churches in rural areas provide a major avenue for keeping elders meaningfully involved in their community. Having access to this resource requires establishing communication with the ministers of these churches.

We have also found that ministers can be extremely helpful adjuncts in therapy. For example, one minister recently assisted us with an older woman who had a recurring history of admissions to the state hospital for depression. Each time a depressive episode occurred, the woman got angry and wanted to do harm to the people around her; she took this as evidence that she was being influenced by the devil. The woman was extremely passive and never expressed anger, even though there were numerous occasions in her life when it would have been appropriate. In therapy sessions we were unable to effectively counter her beliefs about the devil or work on getting the woman to express her anger in more productive ways. Because we did not share her religious background, she dismissed all of our comments that anger is normal and does not mean possession by the devil. As an alternative course of action and with her permission, we discussed her situation with the minister that she had indicated she liked and greatly admired. Following consultation with us, the minister visited her in her home and told her essentially the same things we had been saying—that anger is normal and does not mean possession by the devil. She arrived at the next therapy session both greatly relieved and ready to work on more productive means of expressing her anger.

To establish this kind of reciprocal consultation, we have set up individual meetings with other service providers, rather than the more efficient alternative of meeting with them in groups, for the following reasons. First of all, as we have outlined elsewhere, the importance in rural areas of personal relationships and informal communication networks is critical. Second, we have found that it is easier for other service providers to discuss difficult situations on a one-to-one basis rather than in front of their peers. In addition to meeting with other service providers on an individual basis, we also feel it is important to convey to other service providers a willingness to share our skills and information as well as a feeling that we can also benefit from their background and experience. We have found that as we show a willingness to consult with them in areas of their expertise, they show an increased willingness to consult with us in areas in which we have more background and experience.

Workshops and meetings. Perhaps one of the most enjoyable forms of nontraditional therapy in which we have engaged is the workshop. Topics have ranged from such highly focalized issues as death and dying to broader issues such as coping with the stresses of aging. Length of the workshops has ranged from a single one-hour session to several all-day sessions over the course of a summer. Meetings have been conducted through community education classes, local organizations, or the sponsorship of the local Area Agency on Aging (these latter workshops were conducted in conjunction with our colleague, Linda S. Davis, Ph.D.). Future sessions are in the planning stages through local churches and for a home health care organization for the aged.

In our view there are many advantages to the workshop format. Perhaps one of the most important advantages of the workshop is its ability to attract people who would find it embarrassing to be seen going for psychological help: not only is there no stigma associated with attending a program that is billed as educational, but it can even be prestigious. Therefore, people who may be having concerns in a particular area can have access to psychologists or other mental health professionals in order to discuss areas of concern without having to come in for "therapy." We have found that many people will feel that the information provided in the workshop is sufficient to answer their concerns. Others may phone us for additional information or meetings, and still others may use the workshops as a first step on the way to seeking out individual help in a traditional therapy format.

A second advantage of the workshop format is that people who want information but wish to remain anonymous can do so. Some individuals who would never ask specifically for help for themselves can sit quietly, take whatever skills and strategies are provided, and go home to try them without ever having had to make public that they have a concern. However, we typically find that these same people often open up by the end of the workshop, after realizing that many of their peers have very similar problems and that others are willing to voice their concerns with no aversive consequences. However, the anonymity they expect before coming seems to be an important factor in attracting them to the workshops in the first place.

A third advantage of the workshop format relates to the number and type of people reached. The workshops we present are designed not only for the aged, but for their families and for others who provide services to the aged such as ministers, social workers, workers in senior centers, agriculture extension agents, van drivers, workers with Meals-on-Wheels, etc. Since older people themselves are less likely to seek out psychological services, our rationale has been to work with the younger people with whom they have contact who are more willing to seek out information and help in these areas. We also feel that this approach has distinct advantages over traditional therapy approaches in that it utilizes natural support systems in the elders' environments. According to unpublished research that we have recently completed, friends and members of the family are the people to whom elders most prefer to turn when they have concerns. In addition, these people have contact with the elders on a day-to-day basis. It seems to us, then, that the more enduring approach is to take advantage of those resource persons who already exist in the elders' environments. These persons can not only assist the elders with their concerns, but will have an advantage in dealing with similar concerns when they arise in their own lives.

A fourth advantage to the workshop format is that it is an efficient means of disseminating information. Given that so many people in rural areas have unmet needs, the traditional one-to-one therapy situation may for some purposes be unnecessarily cumbersome. In workshops, much of the same information can be conveyed that would be included in a traditional therapy approach and the time of the presenter is maximized by sharing with many people at once.

A fifth advantage of workshops is that they are presented as education and participants have no qualms if they are not expected to pay. In our culture, educational programs are already seen as being earned through taxes and as being a right rather than a service. Elders, therefore, do not have an expectation that they should pay for such services, and those with limited financial resources can take advantage of them.

A final advantage to the workshop is that the participants in the workshop have often already encountered many of the problems that are discussed. This has a variety of positive features. One is that other participants can often serve as excellent role models when they relate the ways in which they have successfully dealt with particular problems. Also, in discussing their concerns participants convey that it is acceptable to have problems and to voice them and ask for assistance. In addition, the participants can serve as excellent sources of information for each other; often some are aware of resources in the community or techniques of handling problems that can be very useful to the others. An additional advantage is that participants can greatly enhance the credibility of those who are conducting the workshops. It is much more likely that workshop participants will try suggestions if other participants indicate that a given approach worked for them.

Setting up workshops that appeal. In setting up workshops a number of issues are encountered that need to be considered if the workshops are to attract participants and function effectively. The first of these is the selection of a location that is relatively central to the people who are expected to attend, that does not require driving on difficult, heavily traveled roads during peak traffic times, and that has adequate, easily accessible parking areas. Selection of a location that does not require climbing flights of stairs, that has adequate furniture (most elementary schools would be inappropriate unless furnished to handle adults as well), and that has easily accessible bathrooms is also critical. If meetings are to be held in the evenings, the area should be well lit. On different occasions, we have used high school and college classrooms, a university conference center, and the meeting rooms in churches, banks, and restaurants. In announcing the location, we have found that clearly drawn maps showing how to find the workshop should be included in the fliers. Major routes in and out, special landmarks, and places to park should all be clearly illustrated. Such a provision is likely to attract people who live farther away or are less familiar with the community.

The time of day that the workshop is scheduled is also important. In order to attract elders, midmorning through midafternoon seems to be the best choice, because this period avoids the worst traffic hours and does not require night driving. Because of work schedules, weekday evenings and weekends are the best times for the families of elders. However, the topic must be unusually attractive in order to get them to attend even at these times. If the workshop is aimed at those who work with the elderly, weekdays seem to be preferred, as attendance can often then be arranged as part of their jobs. Because of the varying needs, workshops will have to be scheduled to be most convenient to whichever audience you are working hardest to attract. Scheduling will, of course, have to conform as well to the availability of meeting areas (schools, for example, are not available in the daytime) and to the modes of transportation available.

A third issue in rural areas is transportation. We have found that the following considerations can improve attendance. First, if there is a volunteer service organization in the community, its members may be willing to set up car pools to bring in elders from outlying towns and counties. Similarly, rides can often be obtained by making requests through church bulletins or by announcements from pastors. In some communities it may be possible to use a church or school bus by paying a fee to the driver; if at all possible, the workshop sponsors rather than the participants should absorb this cost, because it might pose a hardship for those wishing to attend. If an effort is to be made to provide transportation, it is important to make arrangements in the early planning states, so that potential participants can be notified of the existence of rides at the same time that they are informed that the workshop will occur.

Advertising the workshops is a fourth issue. We have advertised workshops through a variety of means—direct mailings to anyone in the community that we know has an interest in aging (the local Area Agency on Aging maintains a list of all people in the area who provide any kind of services to the aged), announcements in supermarkets and laundromats, and advertisements in church bulletins. Local radio and television stations have carried announcements as public service bulletins, and workshops have been listed in upcoming events columns in local newspapers. We have also found that word of mouth from previous workshop participants is an important way to advertise, and we routinely mail announcements to anyone who has previously participated in a workshop.

A fifth issue is the selection of a topic. The topic must, of course, deal with an issue that presents problems for older people, but beyond that it is quite open. Our presentations have covered independence skills (driving, medications, living arrangements, etc.); assertiveness skills (how to really tell your elderly parents/adult children what you want them to know, how to say "no" to a salesman, how to get a bureaucracy like the phone company to treat you fairly, etc.); how to make the most of retirement; sexuality and aging; dealing with death (writing a will with or without a lawyer, dealing with the loss of a spouse and of friends, nursing a chronically ill person at home, etc.); and simply what changes can be expected with age and how to cope with them.

Making the workshops therapeutic. After the initial planning stages have been completed, the remaining problem is to structure the workshops so that they can be a form of therapy. We have found that there are several features that should be incorporated into a workshop if it is to serve this function.

The first feature relates to the way in which information is to be presented. While theoretical information and statistics can be interesting, it has been our experience that this kind of information is best kept to a minimum. This kind of content has value, but only if it is followed by information on how it can be put to practical use. As much as possible, therefore, the content of the workshop should provide practical information on how to deal with problems that are likely to arise. It is important to be concrete and provide numerous examples, since abstractions and generalities are difficult to use. For instance, we point out that it is important for people of all ages to make as many of their own choices as possible, and that making choices is possible in nearly every situation. We use as illustrations the more difficult situations that may come up. For example, if it has been determined that an elderly person must enter a nursing home, the elder can still exercise some choice by being told about the facilities that exist, visiting them, and being allowed to select among them.

In addition to presenting practical information, we have found that the information seems to elicit more response if it is supplemented by role-playing or demonstrations rather than through a straight lecture format. We found in one workshop on family relationships, for example, that as we described how to tell a spouse firmly, gently, caringly, and honestly about one's feelings we were met by quiet, polite listening. However, when we supplemented this by acting out scenes in which a wife and her recently retired husband encountered and solved problems in adjusting to their new life situation, we were confronted with a barrage of questions on how to deal with other situations. Such demonstrations also provide concrete examples of how to apply techniques that have previously been discussed, so there is less chance that they are misunderstood and incorrectly applied.

In addition to using role-playing and demonstrations, we have found that a lot of response can be generated if some of the information is provided by elders who have encountered and coped with particular situations. Not only does this mean that other elders at the workshop acquire information from a peer and will therefore trust that the advice works, but the experience can also be therapeutic for the person who has been asked to speak, in that it provides him or her with the opportunity to help others. Some of the best-received presentations at our workshops have been by a 70-year-old retired railroad worker who discussed his strategies for preparing for retirement and listed what he'd determined had been the most and least effective; by an 81-year-old practical nurse who discussed her philosophy of helping and happiness after 65; by a 60-year-old county employee who discussed how she had assisted her elderly clients in becoming more active; and by a 72-year-old president of a chapter of the American Association of Retired Persons who described in detail how he and several other people had set up that chapter with suggestions to others on what should be considered in starting and maintaining new interest groups.

Another feature that we have found important to incorporate into workshops is the opportunity for small group discussions. In part this is important because the variety in format serves to maintain interest. However, the primary importance of these discussions is that they give participants the opportunity to talk about personal concerns regarding themselves or aged members of their families. In structuring these discussions, we begin by asking group members to accomplish a specific task—for example, generating ways to ease the transition into retirement. This is used as a point of departure to get group members to begin talking. In addition, we try to arrange the groups so that they are composed of both younger and older members. This allows group members to look at an issue from a variety of different perspectives and allows older and younger members to serve as resources for each other. Also, we feel it is important for each group to be led by one of those conducting the workshop in order to facilitate group interaction. We feel our function in leading the small groups is to encourage group members to interact with each other, rather than to serve in the role of expert.

The groups can serve a variety of therapeutic functions. For example, during one of these groups, the topic of discussion included placing older parents in nursing homes. During this discussion, one older woman related the difficulties she had encountered in placing her husband in a nursing home and making sure that he had adequate care. For this woman, the small group both provided a source of sympathy and support and resulted in information from another older group member on a different nursing home of comparable cost where the level of care was much better. For younger participants this group provided the opportunity to get firsthand information on the emotional and financial difficulties involved in such a decision.

Another feature to enhance the therapeutic function of the workshops is to provide frequent breaks and to remain easily accessible during these breaks. We view such breaks not as an opportunity to rest, but as an opportunity for others to approach us with issues or concerns that have arisen during the workshop. We have found that a great deal of therapy can be accomplished near the water fountain, over lunch, and even in the restrooms. Many of the people in our audiences will save personal questions for those times, and it is often those questions that they most want to have answered. During breaks we have been asked such questions as how to cope with a dying husband's needs, personal concerns about sexuality, and how to deal with an older family member who is becoming senile.

However, even break times are too public for some, and we have made a point of making clear to workshop participants how they can contact us at a later time if they wish to. We have often found that after a workshop we are subsequently contacted by several of the participants.

We have encountered numerous examples of the therapeutic effects of the workshops. Some of these effects occur for people who attend the workshops and may never speak up or ask a question. For example, we heard from the husband of a woman who had participated in one of our workshops on coping with physical changes in old age. The husband described his wife as having become increasingly despondent over the last couple of years as she began to notice changes in her sensory and motor abilities, and interpreted these to mean that she was no longer capable. He informed us that the workshops had been instrumental in lifting her depression and getting her to be actively involved in her community once again.

In other situations, workshop participants have been quiet during the sessions and then called us later for additional information. For example, after one workshop on maximizing independence for elders, we were contacted by a woman who described the difficulties she had been experiencing since her mother had been forced to come and live with her. She and her mother were in frequent conflict because she felt her mother should not be doing anything around the house and should instead sit down and be taken care of. Her mother, on the other hand, would often try to do chores that were far too difficult for her, given her state of health. She informed us that following the workshop she realized the importance to her mother of maintaining as much of her independence as possible, and she made arrangements to meet with us later to discuss how she could go about sitting down with her mother to work out an arrangement that allowed the mother to do as much as possible for herself while still not doing chores that would worsen her condition.

The reception that our workshops have received has generally been excellent. Participants have made a point of staying after the workshops to convey to us how valuable they felt they were and frequently contact us to find out when future workshops will be held.

Nontraditional groups. Our third nontraditional approach in providing psychological services to the aged has been through setting up group experiences for elders. In setting up a group, the first problem we encountered was how to structure the group to make it acceptable to potential participants. It was our feeling that labeling the group a "therapy" group would have attached a stigma that would have prevented the group from ever being formed. It would also have set up expectations of therapy as it is traditionally conceived, which would have narrowed the scope of the group as we wished to offer it. We therefore decided to describe our group as having three purposes not typically associated with therapy.

Our first purpose was to serve as an information source for group members, offering information typically unavailable to rural elders. For instance, information about services in the community would include types of medical care available, how to qualify for Medicare and Medicaid, housing specifically designed to meet the needs of elders, service agencies available, stores which offer specials for elders, etc. It was also anticipated that group members would serve as important information sources for each other. Interaction among group members would additionally point out areas for which we had no information immediately available. We hoped this would get group members interested in becoming involved with gathering and sharing that material within the group.

Our second purpose was to assist elders in increasing their skills in coping with the many problems associated with aging. By focusing on communication, problem-solving, and preparations for foreseeable events, we hoped to enhance physical and psychological adjustment for both the present and future without focusing on individual dynamics or personality analysis.

Our third purpose was to have the participants teach us about the problems encountered in growing old and how they dealt with them. We saw this not only as a learning experience for the facilitators, but also as a therapeutic benefit for the participants through knowing they were contributing to others and were "earning" the services that they received. We decided to make it clear that we were meeting with the group in order to share in the learning rather than to "do" something to the members. Our role was to be that of facilitator, not expert, and our task was to help the members help each other.

As has been stated earlier, attempting to make contact with rural elders has certain obstacles not found in urban settings. Contacts are not made through conventional channels but rather through personal acquaintance or favorable recommendations. Therefore, when attempting to establish our first group we were faced with inevitable problems in obtaining group members.

The first problem was one of determining the most efficient means of making contact with the elder population. It was decided that going through an organization which had regular contact with older persons would enhance the possibilities of obtaining a sufficient number of persons to set up an effective group. In an attempt to attract a diverse group we limited our contacts to two organizations which dealt with a wide variety of persons. The two contacts served to reaffirm our previous conclusions about the necessity of constructing a network of associations within the community.

The first attempt, with an organization devoted to keeping elders in contact with each other through social means, never got past the initial appeal. Our calls were not returned and the persons with whom we spoke were not receptive to us in any way. The disinterest (and possibly distrust) was total; we were simply ignored. The second contact was with an organization offering the possibility of volunteer service by and for elderly persons. The director had had previous contact with us under other circumstances and was immediately open to discuss our plans. Although there were reservations, we quickly elicited a commitment for a hearing. The person with whom we spoke made direct reference to our established credibility and stated that time would be made for us because of the quality of our prior relationship.

Our conversations with the director of this organization included some carefully thought-out information. We explained the purpose of the group in detail, focusing on the benefits to the members. In addition, we pointed out ways in which the group would benefit the goals of the organization by enhancing members' abilities to cope, help each other, and make better use of their skills. We also touched on the fact that participation by members of the organization would help others by allowing us to collect information and disseminate it to professionals and lay persons. The emphasis was on helping, not on therapy, and the appeal was made with an intent of mutual achievement. Again, we did not take the expert role, but attempted to set up a working relationship based on equal gain. In turn, the director approached the organization's members with the same attitude and was met with a positive, though hesitant, response from several members.

Although the organization's director based the appeal for members on the criteria provided by us, we are certain that the immediate response by the elders themselves was based on trust and expectations already existing in that organization. By working through established channels we were thus able to capitalize on longstanding rapport and begin our contact under the halo effect of that relationship. Had we attempted to make contact directly, the project would have proceeded far more slowly. Having an accepted community member voice our ideas gave them a credibility which would otherwise have been difficult to achieve.

Our second problem was a direct consequence of working in a rural area. This problem was the selection and screening of group members. By virtue of the fact that we were working in an area with reduced population density, the range of potential participants from whom we could draw was greatly reduced, and we therefore had much less control over the heterogeneity or homogeneity of the group. Because of the smaller population and current life expectancies we anticipated having a majority of women. However, if we did obtain male group members we were concerned, since traditional sex roles predominate in elder cohorts, that there might be reduced openness and spontaneity in a mixed group. Of equal concern was our determination to work with people as they were available in the community and not to place artificial restrictions on our group's makeup, in which case a mix of males and females would be an appropriate membership, despite the potential problems. We opted for a wait-and-see approach, with the attitude that we would attempt to overcome obstacles of sex distribution or communication problems as they arose, perhaps making them a discussion topic for the group.

Screening in relation to race caused multiple concerns. The population from whom we would be drawing is white, Mexican-American, and black in a roughly 70:20:10 percent distribution. Not only were we aware of the fact that our group members were likely to have had little or no previous social contact with persons of other races—our area being a part of the Deep South tradition—we were also concerned about the problems inherent in convening a group with persons of sharply differing cultural and language backgrounds. There was a real possibility that unless we screened for race we would acquire group members with radically diverse values, modes of social interaction, and English language skills, who had virtually no understanding of others' life-styles. In that case, group cohesion would be seriously jeopardized. However, after weighing the issue we again decided to adopt a wait-and-see attitude. We prepared to deal with the issue of differences within the group as they became apparent. Parenthetically, let us state that we have as yet found no effective way of drawing participation from the Mexican-American population. Language and cultural differences seem to discriminate strongly against our appealing to those elders. We hypothesize that contacts are best made by Spanish-speaking persons who have already established credibility with the Mexican-American subgroup.

Getting the new group off the ground. Our first group consisted of ten women, four black and six white. They ranged in age from 65 to 88 and cut across all socioeconomic levels. Attending members were tentative about their participation in the group, voicing some confusion about its purpose. Most reported that they had come on the recommendation of the organization's director and would not have come otherwise. However, once there, they were receptive to us and willing to listen to what we had to offer.

The first session began with introductions. We told the members who we were and how we happened to be involved in the group. We presented the purposes and how they might relate to each person individually. Members were offered an opportunity to introduce themselves and interact briefly. We then stated our intentions for "ground rules" covering attendance, confidentiality, participation, etc. After a short discussion, members contracted to meet for four weeks, with negotiation for continuing four-week periods at that time.

The last part of the meeting was devoted to members and leaders socializing over coffee. Meeting time was placed at one-and-a-half hours each week, in the morning when everyone felt fresh (at a later point we found it necessary to reduce the length of the meetings because the group members became visibly tired after one hour).

During the first session several interesting aspects of the members' interactions became apparent. We discovered that members introduced themselves and conversed in a formal manner, addressing each other as "Miss" or "Mrs." Members did not carry on discussion without encouragement and looked to the leaders to direct the proceedings. There was little spontaneous responding and no self-disclosure. It was evident that they wished to know in advance what was coming and that structure would be necessary. Even during the social time members were very formal.

It also became apparent at the first meeting that group members varied widely in level of physical functioning, autonomy, availability of support groups, socioeconomic level, and past experience. Differences were blatantly obvious, some of which had to be dealt with immediately. One member, for instance, had a significant hearing loss, which necessitated changing the seating arrangement to insure her full participation in subsequent meetings. We audio-taped each session and had a leaders' meeting after each session in which we reviewed the audio tape and discussed changes to be made and plans for future sessions. We found these meetings to be extremely important for successful functioning of the group.

In the second group meeting we introduced a relevant topic for discussion. Such a structured beginning served several useful purposes. First, it served as an icebreaker for the members and provided them an opportunity to see what was expected of them. Members new to a group situation are often anxious about disclosing themselves, and the discussion of a topic of mutual interest can serve as a means by which individuals learn to participate and self-disclose. If the topic is chosen well, the members will begin to relate their own experiences and feelings, and the leaders and other members can begin to learn about them and their lives. For example, a discussion about the financial problems associated with growing old drew a spirited discussion in this initial group session, and several members went into detail about their monetary difficulties. Thus, a norm for self-disclosure was established, and a feeling of commonality began immediately to grow among members. Other topics of interest to serve this function in a budding group might include the changing relationship between the elderly person and his or her children, inactivity in retirement, loss of autonomy, etc. The topics to be discussed need only be relevant and relatively nonthreatening—death and dying is probably too sensitive an issue with which to begin.

After the second group meeting, members began to interact in a more relaxed manner, although they still referred to each in formal terms. They did seem comfortable calling the leaders by their first names, a fact which we took to be a reflection of the increased comfort with the group experience. We continued to offer a general topic of discussion for each session, but members began to mold those topics to fit their own needs and circumstances. For instance, a session which began with a general discussion on preparation and safety of personal papers became the basis for a two-session exploration of the need for and proper making of wills and funeral arrangements. Members shared experiences, feelings, and how-to's on an increasing basis and began to express relief at having others with whom they could openly converse about these matters. One member who had rapidly failing health was concerned that after her death her possessions would be distributed without her consent, yet she did not have the finances to retain an attorney and draw up a will. Through discussion with the group and legal information provided by a volunteer in the legal profession, our member executed a legal will, using a standard form which is available in this state, and filed it with the county clerk. Without the group she would most probably have remained anxious and unprotected for the rest of her life. Group support and information relieved her of those burdens.

Other topic areas were included throughout the life of the group on problems of loss of independence, preparation for deterioration of health, ways of dealing with loss of friends and family, general problems of living alone, and financial management. Still other information included services and aids for the elderly available on a local, statewide, and national basis.

The fourth meeting came and went with members enthusiastically renewing the contract to meet. Comments about the increasing importance of the group began to be heard on a regular basis. As we had hoped, members began checking on each other and expressing concern for those unable to attend at different times. Interest in new activities and information was generated, and members shared such diverse knowledge as which stores offered discounts to older persons and how to change sheets on a bed without all the usual lifting and pulling.

Techniques that proved successful. Later meetings were devoted to focusing on topics initiated by members. We discovered that problem-solving skills of the members tended to be inefficient. Based on that information, we introduced a method of problem solving. The approach we found most useful is outlined in *Clinical Behavior*

Therapy (Goldfried and Davison, 1976). Briefly, the approach is divided into four steps: (1) the problem is identified and clarified; (2) a brainstorming session is used to generate all possible alternative solutions to the problem under discussion; (3) the alternatives are evaluated for their possible utility; and (4) the individual tries various alternatives that seem most useful.

We found that many problems associated with aging were bewildering and threatening to our members. As their social contacts dwindled, the feedback and information that went with these contacts decreased. Opportunities to learn new methods of solving their problems diminished, often leaving them with outdated or inappropriate coping skills. The group offered a forum for practicing problem-solving steps which they could use outside the group. The method was used on several occasions when members stated a complaint or worry and were unable to pinpoint their exact problem or useful solutions. For example, one member had limited transportation and was becoming increasingly isolated. Members brainstormed and constructed a list of fourteen possible ways of increasing contacts. Emphasis was placed on number of alternatives produced, and seemingly far-fetched or unusual responses were encouraged. Among the ideas were doing phone visiting with shut-ins on a daily basis, "housesitting" for those on vacation, beginning an exploration of areas within walking distance, joining a church or doing volunteer work for organizations which offer transportation, and getting into a hot meals program which also has a ride service for elderly persons. Other suggestions centered around neighborhood activities and were very clever and innovative. Members were excited and pleased to find that they were able to generate many possibilities in a very short period of time. The individual member began to act on the alternatives presented and shortly thereafter reported a new sense of involvement and worth as a participating member of the community.

Another technique found useful was behavioral contracting. As Stuart (1977) states in *Behavioral Self-Management,* the limits of the behavioral contract are only those of client sophistication and level of rapport with the therapist. Therefore, contracts can be as elementary or complex as the individual situation warrants. For example, early in the project we established an informal contract with the group to meet for four weeks with absences only in case of absolute necessity. In later sessions, specific contracts that were carefully written out and signed were successfully used to change behavior. For example, one overweight member wished to "have more energy." To arrive at behavioral goals the group engaged in the problem-solving technique discussed earlier. Three target behaviors were selected: (1) participating in an exercise program (walking a specified distance each day); (2) eating at specified times each day; and (3) eating slowly and thoroughly (by chewing each bite to liquid and putting eating utensils down between each bite). The group witnessed the drawing up of the contract and the signing of the document. Times, increases in activities, and rewards and punishments were specified. During subsequent meetings the first order of business for the group was to inquire about this and other contracts, and time was devoted to social reinforcement or comment about failures. Within three weeks the member began to report success in adhering to the contract, losing weight, and increasing her energy level. Within five weeks she reported a weight loss of twelve pounds and increased her walking range from two blocks once a day to fourteen blocks twice a day.

A third technique applied successfully in the group was rational restructuring, as outlined in *Reason and Emotion in Psychotherapy* (Ellis, 1962). This technique is based on the premise that irrational assumptions are the direct cause of emotional discomfort, and that restructuring faulty cognitions will lead to healthier emotional responses. We used the technique any time we engaged the group in discussing the usefulness and logic of a member's attitudes, beliefs, and methods of coping. In one instance a member with deteriorating health described her increasing anxiety about her diminishing ability to live a worthwhile life. When asked about her support group, she told us she could not bring herself to request help from her children or neighbors because of her humiliation at being a "helpless old lady." Further discussion revealed that she felt that persons who are not totally autonomous are essentially worthless. We elicited responses from the group members and engaged in a discussion about the logic of her assumptions. Other individuals quickly confronted the person with examples of how her assumptions were not functional. The specific self-statements that the woman was making were detailed, and more functional substitutes suggested. She then contracted to practice saying the new statements instead of the old and to begin asking for help with specific activities. In later sessions members continued to check on her progress. The combination of group support and confrontation gave a safe, structured method of establishing a new mode of coping.

Assertiveness was never a formal topic in the group, but virtually every session offered an opportunity for training on an informal basis. Several members expressed some situationally specific lack of assertiveness, and members were encouraged to practice new behaviors through role-play and role-rehearsal. One member in particular benefited from the opportunity to explore her rights and responsibilities. A highly religious person, this black woman was constantly at the beck and call of anyone who wished to ask for help. Her submissiveness was based on a belief that she must love and serve all persons in order to be a good member of her religion. The resulting selflessness was leading her to deny her own needs and wants and consequently to suffer seriously deteriorating health. In discussing the problem with her, we pointed out that if all persons are to be loved and served equally, our member herself must be served, and that meant self-care. The idea that she could, and in fact "should" (according to her values) say "no" to others and allow herself some privacy and rest was a revelation to our member. She contracted to keep one day each week totally clear for herself, and, after practicing assertive responding with other members, established a pattern of saying "no" with a clear conscience. Six months after the group ended she was still being assertive about her time and was guilt-free for the first time in 50 years.

Outcomes of the group were positive in many dimensions. Members became more open, more involved in each other, less isolated, and better able to control their lives. Many of them commented on a new realization of the joy of living. Others reported a much reduced feeling of hopelessness. Practical, day-to-day problems were solved as members explored alternatives together, and certainly the leaders' abilities were enriched as a result of the experience.

As we terminated our meetings, the organization's director contacted us with a request for other groups. She reported that members had been emphatic in their positive response to the group and had asked to be included in further activities of that type. In addition, other members of the organization had requested that they be included in any new group that might be formed. The enthusiastic response leads us to believe that the format we have used is an effective service-delivery method that can be duplicated in other communities. Subsequent experience with similar groups has reinforced our use of these techniques and ways of viewing the problems that confront elderly persons.

Summary

We have attempted to provide psychological services to rural elders both by trying to make traditional avenues of therapy more accessible and through the less traditional modes of reciprocal consultation with other service providers, workshops, and group experiences. We have found all of these approaches to be useful, although each approach requires as a first step the gradual process of establishing informal personal relationships with others in the community. We have continually found that once the initial barriers are overcome, all of these approaches have been received enthusiastically.

6

Facilitating the Transition to Nursing Homes

Carol J. Dye and Cherryl C. Richards

The transition from home into nursing home can be one of the most difficult of life's adjustments. This may be so for a number of reasons. One of the most important of these has to do with the meaning of this transition. In entering the nursing home, the individual must relinquish many of the possessions and cease many of the activities that have been important throughout life. Consequently, the nursing home often is perceived as the last residence the individual will have (Atchley, 1972; Butler & Lewis, 1977; Kalish, 1975). It is the end of the road. Moreover, this transition often is precipitated by some physical incapacity and comes at a time when physical energies are normally on the wane. Therefore the individual has reduced energies with which to cope with adjustment to the change itself.

The negative effects of nursing home placement have been seen not only in an increase in death rate (Aldrich & Mendkoff, 1963; Blenkner, 1967; Jasnau, 1967; Lieberman, 1961) but also in the area of psychological functioning (Lieberman, 1969; Lieberman, Prock, and Tobin, 1968). With the onset of the social, physical, and mental traumas that may accompany aging, the individual's self-concept begins to decline. Then, if institutionalization is necessary, a meaningful blow is dealt to the declining self-concept. Those who have worked with the elderly have indicated that women in particular react to being institutionalized as an indication of being unloved and rejected by their family. In addition, those who survive in the institutional environment for any length of time react adversely, that is, they become disoriented to time and place and show increased preoccupation with body and lowered emotional responsivity (Lieberman and Lakin, 1963; Morris, 1975).

While studies and experience with older adults demonstrate that the transition to a nursing home can be difficult, little seems to have been done to find ways of preparing the older adult for institutional life. Markus et al. (1972) proposed that the elderly individual be screened more fully before placement to avoid lack of congruence between himself and his environment. The authors suggested that this preplacement screening might help to reduce some of the adjustment problems that might arise during placement. In her discussion of social work services within the long-term care facility, Brody (1974) indicated the need to help the older adult at several points in the placement process—during the waiting period, during the period of admission, and immediately after admission.

Screening and counseling at all the steps along the way to placement, as Brody indicated, might be advantageous for both the older adults and their families. Counseling regarding the perceived and actual necessity of nursing home placement of older relatives would seem to be of undoubted benefit to everyone concerned, allowing the entire family to explore the basis for placement, the problems, and the feelings involved. This type of counseling would encourage support and understanding between the older adult and those who are important in making the decision for the placement. Discussion of the appropriate nursing home to best fit the individual's need could take place. Counseling during and after the time of placement could also be beneficial for the aged and for their families. This would provide an opportunity to explore feelings, ask questions, and express doubts and fears at each of these points in the process. In this counseling the older adult might be able to gain support in making necessary adjustments.

Finding ways of facilitating the adjustment of moving from one's own home into the nursing home environment through counseling and other procedures was the focus of a research project funded through the National Institute on Aging (evaluation of these procedures is in progress). Two similar group procedures were developed. One of these was a series of group counseling sessions for elderly individuals newly admitted to a nursing home, hereafter called the *resident group.* These groups were composed of from three to seven members. It was necessary to keep the number of people in a group small since it was difficult to provide an opportunity for all to participate fully with more present. Older adults, especially frail elderly, seem to respond better in smaller groups. They seem to prefer discussing issues on a one-to-one basis rather than focusing on the total number of persons in a group. The experience with these groups was that even a group of three moderately verbal older adults can be sufficient and result in the appropriate group process.

The other series of group meetings involved elderly people newly admitted to the nursing home plus family members who were important in making the decision for placement. This was the *family group.* Generally no more than five family units could be included in one of these groups. With the older adult and one family member this would make ten people in the group. Again, at least three older adults and their families would be necessary to keep the group intact.

The older adults who were selected for participation in these groups had to be at a level of mental alertness that would allow them to contribute to the group and also to be able to gain from the group process. They also had to have at least moderately intact verbal skills. While these were the general criteria, some individuals who were considered confused were also included for participation. These individuals didn't know what the date was, who they were, where they were, or other particulars about their environment. Yet these individuals experienced and could express the same feelings about loneliness, separation, and vulnerability that the more lucid members of our group had and could relate.

Newly admitted residents were selected for participation since they were still actively in the process of adjustment to the transition. The group meetings had a specific purpose, i.e., to discuss the problems involved in entering a nursing home, and were time limited, i.e., they were scheduled for a certain number of sessions. These two factors were thought to be important in motivating elderly persons to participate. Older adults, especially those who are just entering nursing homes, are concerned with conservation of their energies. They seem to be more likely to invest those energies in activities that are specific and relevant to their own needs and in those that do not require an extended commitment.

Rationale for Group Counseling

The rationale for developing this method of assisting in the adjustment process was that group meetings would allow older adults and their families a chance to discuss their feelings and concerns about placement and to find ways to solve some of the concomitant problems. The resident group was developed to help participants gain support from each other. The family group was designed to create closer family ties. The goal was to increase understanding between the older adult and his family so that an integrated family unit could provide emotional support for one another beyond the time of the group sessions.

Those coming from their own homes into the nursing home were chosen to participate in this study because of the special problems they might have. Individuals coming from the hospital into the nursing home were likely to have been told by their doctor that they needed nursing home care. The fact of the hospitalization and the suggestion of an authority (the doctor) may demonstrate to the individual that he is unable to care for himself and might make accepting nursing home placement less difficult. Those who come from one nursing home into another are already somewhere along in the adjustment process. By comparison, moving from home to nursing home may be the most difficult of these transitions because of lingering doubts regarding the ability to care for oneself, whether this was the right time and decision, whether other alternatives to placement might have been tried, etc. The rationale for providing counseling *after* placement in the nursing home rather than *before* was that inquiries of nursing homes revealed that placement is a precipitous event. Contrary to the expectations from the reports in the literature that older adults wait for admission to nursing homes sometimes up to a year, it was the experience in setting up these groups that not much time elapsed between the decision for placement and the actual event. In addition, there really was not an effective way to locate people who were in the process of making this decision. Families could be identified when they began to call nursing homes, but placement tended to take place within a few days, leaving little or no time for counseling. Possibly those situations in which there is a long wait before admission are those in which a particular home is preferred and the older adult is still minimally capable of sustaining himself in the community and therefore is not in immediate need of placement.

Both the resident and the family group sessions were scheduled for seven meetings of approximately an hour's duration each session. These seven sessions were called a "workshop" to avoid any problems in resistance that there might be to the notion of counseling or therapy. The seven sessions were conducted by two clinical psychologists. This was mentioned in the group in the first session in order to promote an honest relationship. The leaders of the group introduced themselves as Doctors ______ and ______ and all the particulars of the study were related once again to be certain that the older adults would know why they were there and what was to be accomplished. From this point on, however, titles and position were not mentioned unless brought up by the group members. In order to facilitate a relaxed and giving atmosphere, the leaders expressed the desire to be called by their first names. The older adults were called by their preferred names.

The sequence of the sessions was the same for both the resident and the family groups. The first meeting was planned as an introductory session. The second, third, and fourth sessions were planned to center around the feelings and concerns about placement. The discussions in sessions five and six were to be concerned with solving some of the problems that arose in the nursing home. The last session was the concluding or wrap-up session.

There were several objectives for those who participated in the workshops. One objective was to help the older adult form supportive attachments since separation, loneliness, and isolation were seen to be important problems in placement. This was to be done by helping the older adults form friendships with other older adults and by reinforcing positive existing relationships within the family groups. Another objective was to help these older adults to explore and discuss their concerns and to share and help resolve their feelings regarding the change in life-style that came with entrance into the nursing home. A third objective was to help the older adult become aware of feelings toward those who were involved in making the decision for nursing home placement and determine ways of dealing with those feelings. A fourth objective was to discuss alternative ways of solving the problems that arise in institutional living and to try these solutions whenever possible.

In the resident group these objectives were attained by helping the older adult to gain support from the other group members. These older adults were encouraged to learn each others' names and the location of the rooms of the other group members so that they could seek each other out between group sessions. In the family group the objectives were attained by helping the older adult gain support from the other newly admitted residents to the nursing home in the group and by helping the members of the family unit to improve communication and increase understanding of one another. With the family group, the aim was to help all individuals to appreciate the daily problems faced by each person—those experienced both by the aged nursing home resident in adjusting to the nursing home and by the relative, who had many feelings regarding the placement and who had to find ways to show continued support, love, and concern for the older relative. Placement of an older person often means that a relative must find time to visit regularly, furnish small necessities, and help solve the new problems encountered in the home. It is not surprising, then, that realistic considerations of the amount of time involved in coming to the group made it impossible for some families to participate in the family group even though they expressed a great deal of interest and concern for their relative.

Because these have been successful procedures, a greater elaboration and more detailed description of the processes involved, as well as a discussion of the benefits to the elderly person, will follow. Perhaps other nursing home administrators and their staffs would be able to include this group as a regular procedure within their homes. Since the procedure was similar for both the resident and family group they will be discussed together.

Procedures for the Workshop

Session One

The objectives for Session One were to (1) introduce members to one another and become acquainted with one another's names, and (2) help group members become aware of the similarities and differences in the common experience they have had in coming into the nursing home. In this session the leaders took a more active role than in later sessions. The reason for this involvement was that the leaders needed to direct participants in the work of the group and encourage them to share their feelings as fully as possible. The tasks of the first session and the active participation of the leaders allowed group members to begin to establish trust in one another and to feel secure in their relationships within the group. The leaders enhanced this feeling of trust and security by emphasizing that there was a bond of confidentiality between group members regarding what they would relate to one another during the workshop. This bond was necessary in order to enable everyone to speak honestly and freely within the group. Everyone was pledged to this confidence. On the other hand, it was also pointed out that group members could tell other people things of a general nature about the workshop, such as its purpose, without betraying this confidence.

The first task in this session was to have each group member state his/her name. The elderly group members were encouraged to remember the names of the other older adults in the group even though they often protested that their memories were poor. Associations to names were brought to mind and quite a lot of discussion of the names and associations to names was encouraged in this first session. Knowing the names of friends, rather than just recognizing faces, is extremely important in order to establish a greater feeling of attachment. Being able to remember is of equal importance in improving one's self-image. A particular case that supports this belief involved a lady who came to the sessions saying that she couldn't remember anything. In addition, she made other comments indicating generally low self-esteem. After much encouragement and being involved in rehearsing the names of the group members, she was able to remember the names of the members of the group. Her enthusiasm increased and her self-esteem improved visibly. Her newfound ability generalized outside of the group, too. The staff in the home commented to the leaders of the group that this lady seemed to be better able to remember a lot of things since she had been participating in the group. In another instance, group members worked hard in the initial session to learn each others' names. By the fifth session everyone was finally able to recall everyone else's name. As the last person named everyone there was a long pause while the ladies looked around the group and felt quite proud of themselves. Their good feelings were obvious.

The processes involved in this simple Name Game were designed to be generalized beyond remembering names. Attention was given to remembering other things during the group sessions, such as the name of the nursing home or a room number. Ways of remembering things more effectively were given emphasis throughout the sessions whenever there was an appropriate opportunity, while the Name Game took some of the time at the beginning and end of each group session.

After the Name Game was introduced, the process of becoming acquainted with one another was continued by having each older adult relate how he or she happened to come into the nursing home. In the family group also, family members added their perceptions of how this process had occurred. Group members were encouraged to ask questions of each other and the leaders asked questions to bring out some of the feelings that might have been involved. Questions were asked that pertained to the reason for entering the home, what it was like the first day at the home, whether the older adult or his family members had ever been in a nursing home before, whom the person was who was important in making the decision about entering the home, the speed with which the process occurred, and what was left behind, as well as questions relating to some of the feelings about these processes. The importance of preparing the older adult for entrance into a nursing home was stressed by all the group members, as was preparing the family for coping with this situation. The family often expressed the tremendous amount of guilt feelings they suffered when placing their relative in a nursing home. This feeling was often intensified when the older relative expressed the feeling that he/she had been rejected by the family. Often older adults mentioned the feeling of having been dropped off at the nursing home. The family, not knowing the best procedure to follow when faced with this dilemma of placement in a nursing home, may create a very traumatic situation for their older relative. In one extreme and vivid case, the adult children told their aged father they were coming to take him out to dinner. In actuality they did take him out to dinner but then proceeded to "drop" him off at the local nursing home with no explanation. He stood in the lobby totally confused, not knowing where he was. Naturally the reaction was to become hostile not only toward the family but to the nursing home for "keeping" him there against his will.

While members of both family and resident groups related some of the details about placement in Session One, there were often many things left unsaid in this session simply because of lack of time. It wasn't necessary that all details be related since the primary purpose of this first session was to give participants a feeling of being together and sharing in the transition process. The leaders enhanced this process by pointing out the similarities in experience between participants, while they also helped the individuals to relate their own experiences as fully as possible.

After everybody had had a chance to relate some of the things they had experienced during the placement process, Session One was closed with the Name Game so the names and associations newly learned by the older adults at the beginning of the session could be rehearsed. Also, at the end of this session, as well as at the end of each of the next five sessions, some statement was made by the leaders anticipating what might be discussed in the next session. For Session Two, this would be drawn from the content and the process of Session One. Occasionally a group member would have brought up an issue regarding placement that needed to be discussed more fully, or perhaps a thought needed to be elaborated in the next session. Anticipation of the next discussion helped to integrate the workshop meetings and provide continuity between sessions.

Sessions Two, Three, and Four

The objective of these sessions was to explore feelings and concerns about placement. As we worked with these groups of elderly, we found that several issues were of general importance to all. Primary among these were the problems of separation. The feelings resulting from separation from home, family, friends, and pets took up a majority of the time in these three sessions. In addition, there were problems in adjusting to a new living environment, i.e., adjusting to reduced living space, many strangers, and schedules that are not one's own. These were universal problems no matter how much the nursing home staff worked to make the individual feel comfortable.

The move to the nursing home reactivated many feelings of loss previously experienced. There were feelings regarding loss of possessions, of the life-style one pursued, and of the friends and community that was once known. Most of the older adults in these groups had experienced the death of a spouse. That had been an important transition and separation for them that had meant a radical change in life-style and sometimes a move in residence. With entrance into the nursing home almost all of the possessions that had been shared in this life with the spouse became no longer available to them. This was another blow to their ability to cope with the other problems of growing older. Almost always there was sadness expressed regarding the loss of these possessions because of the finality of the situation. All that was left to these older adults were the bare essentials. Sadness was not the only emotion expressed. There was also a good deal of hostility arising over the manner in which their possessions were dispersed. They often indicated how quickly the process had been accomplished, how quickly their things had been sold, etc., and they often expressed the need for more time to prepare for the transition that they had made.

Loss of previously held roles was another part of the separation process. With their entrance into the nursing home, the older adults changed their role from independence to dependence. The role reversal was obvious in some cases. Sometimes an older adult would mistakenly refer to their adult children as "father" or "mother" and then catch themselves in the mistake. This was a good opportunity to get into a discussion of how to maintain self-esteem while coping with increasing dependency.

Many questions arose regarding how to maintain contact with those individuals still left in the community, i.e., family members or those who had been lifelong friends. The need to be able to call or be called on the telephone was mentioned often. Usually some time was spent in each of the groups talking about where the telephone in the home was located and how to find a necessary telephone number. Other means of keeping contact were discussed also. Writing notes or sending cards were mentioned as a difficult process for those with physical disabilities that made it awkward to hold a pen for any period of time. In addition, sending written communications was also made difficult by not having any easy means of obtaining note paper or stamps. These were all problems surrounding the process of separation that involved many feelings and that needed solution.

The order in which these issues and the feelings involved were discussed was not important. They seemed to come up naturally and spontaneously throughout the sessions. The primary job of the leaders of the group during these sessions was to look for the opportunity to explore these more fully, to relate each concern to each group member, and to help each member express feelings regarding these problems. For example, if one group member talked about a pet that had to be left behind, each group member was encouraged to be involved. While not everyone may have left a pet behind, the same process of the severing of ties had occurred at some point in their lives. They could relate to these feelings and give one another support.

Anticipatory perceptions of the nursing home were discussed in every group. Sometimes the leaders asked the group members whether, when they were young, they ever thought they would be in a nursing home. Most times the answer was a definite, emphatic "no." Many of the older adults who participated in these groups indicated that they had cared for their parents as they had grown older and become more disabled and had expected the same for themselves. Sometimes strong feelings of resentment were expressed. At other times the older adults seemed to understand that the changes in life-style from their generation made it necessary for them to enter a nursing home. Another reason for this lack of anticipation was that either they had no experience with nursing homes in their younger years or their experiences had been negative. For example, one gentleman described his perception of a nursing home to be similar to the poor farm near the home of his youth where they put old people out on tethers on a Sunday afternoon. Understandably, these types of images didn't fit what older people had anticipated for their own old age. Whatever the answers to this question, it served to stimulate much discussion regarding the process of placement. A resolution of negative feelings was worked toward by the leaders. The discussion of changes over the generations prompting greater numbers of elderly to enter nursing homes seemed helpful to all group members.

In the family group these sessions provided many opportunities for the sharing of feelings by the members of a family unit and between the members of the various family units. Seeing the similarities with other families often provided greater understanding of one's own situation. In the same ways that the older adult was asked to express his concerns about placement, his relative was also asked. Possibly nothing new was revealed in this interchange, but at times family members learned a great deal about one another.

In the setting of the family group meetings participants had to sit and listen to one another. They could not easily dismiss what the other person had to say or cut one another off. Not only did group members have to listen to one another, the group leaders encouraged them to respond to what was expressed. Everyone was drawn out as to the feelings that might be involved. Group members were encouraged to talk directly to one another. Very often when there is a negative feeling between family members and issues cannot be resolved, they revert to the tactic of talking in the third person about their relative who is present. The group leaders were careful not to allow this to continue and requested family members to address one another directly.

The family group provided the opportunity for the older person to express his feelings about being in a nursing home without being interrupted or cut off by one of his family members. This was clearly demonstrated in one family group where early in the sessions a daughter interrupted her mother frequently to imply that she didn't know what she was talking about. The leaders maintained control and permitted the mother to express her feelings, particularly about separation from her friends and her home, and her feelings about having to remain in the nursing home. Her daughter eventually began to listen and understand her feelings. The mother began to understand and respect her daughter's feelings and they began to develop a new appreciation for each other. When the sessions ended, the daughter stressed several times how much she had gained from the group and how much more cheerful and happier her mother seemed to be. She also indicated that their relationship was now much closer.

One of the things that grew out of these family discussions was a feeling of gratitude and appreciation between family members.

The group leaders worked toward greater expression of these feelings of appreciation. While group members addressed their comments to the group in general, family members were encouraged to talk directly to one another when there was an opportunity to share feelings and especially when there was an expression of understanding or gratitude. Being able to express these feelings was difficult for some people, but when this was accomplished it was tremendously reinforcing for family ties and future support of one another. In one of the family groups, a mother was perceived by her daughter as demanding and ungiving of positive recognition, especially when she attempted to help make her mother comfortable. During the group sessions the necessity for expressing appreciation came up several times and the mother struggled with this. Inwardly, she seemed to know her daughter was working hard for her but she had trouble verbalizing it. By the fifth session she was finally able to verbalize her recognition of her daughter's efforts and the effect on her daughter was quite positive. Not only were the ties between the two strengthened but the effect generalized to other people within the home. The mother was seen to say think you to others for the small things they did for her, whereas before she hadn't been able to do this.

While it was not the purpose of Sessions Two, Three, and Four to find solutions to problems, the need to solve a problem sometimes arose because of the interest of the group or because it seemed like a propitious time for it. Sometimes a small problem, allowing almost immediate solution, was explored. There were questions about medication, food, clothing, contacting family members, being certain about one's finances, etc. These were discussed within the group to determine who else had experienced these problems. Occasionally a group member was given an assignment to try a solution to the problem by the next session. These solutions developed by the group often had to be repeated several times before a member was able to attempt them successfully. As a result problems were sometimes followed for the entire seven sessions.

Sessions Five and Six

In these two sessions group members were more fully directed to the processes of solving problems within the nursing home. Some of these problems were: how to keep track of personal clothing, how to obtain particular kinds of food or modify the way it was prepared or served, how to maintain contact with friends outside, how to contact a relative outside the home, how to keep unwanted, confused persons from wandering into one's room and taking personal possessions, and whom to go to for help.

Group members were encouraged to share feelings, thoughts, and solutions to problems, or to any one problem that could serve as a model for solving other problems. This process of encouraging group members to help one another added to the cohesion of the group. Inevitably, the issue arose concerning how to satisfy needs and yet not appear to be a "complainer." It was quite clear that these older people were concerned that if they asked for too many things perhaps the staff would begin to avoid them. If this were to occur, not only would their needs not be satisfied, their feelings of separation and loneliness would be intensified. As a result, they tended to be quite reticent about solving problems in order to keep this from happening. This problem came up in their relationships with family members as well. Within the context of the family the problem centered around how to ask the help of relatives and convey feelings in such a way that relatives could continue to visit and be of assistance. Support was given among group members that the things being asked about were not undue demands, and that the attitude and the words of the individual doing the inquiring didn't seem to have a complaining quality.

Finding solutions to problems demonstrated to group members that they could achieve something, they could experience success in meeting their needs, they themselves could effect solutions to problems and not always have to rely on others for those solutions. This was especially important in the family group. Often family members outside of the nursing home are relied upon heavily for the coordination of many things for their relative, such as keeping track of laundry done inside the home, medications, supplying small necessities, knowing about schedules, etc. Sometimes visits by relatives become situations in which the older adult waits with a list of things that need to be done and the relative spends the visiting time checking on these things. It is very easy to do too much for those in any type of institution to the point where they are unable to do anything for themselves. They can be overnursed and overcared for into a state of helplessness. When the older adults can do some of these things by themselves, they attain a greater sense of achievement and consequently, their self-esteem improves. In addition, family visits improve in quality and become more relaxing and enjoyable for everyone.

Session Seven

This session was the concluding session, and the leaders became more active again in integrating the group experience for the members so that they could go away from the sessions with some concise idea of what had been discussed, what had been shared, what relationships had been established, and what problem-solving alternatives were discussed during the seven sessions. Much attention was given to those who had made some progress in learning the names of the other members. The ways of remembering by association were again briefly discussed if appropriate. In this session too, an evaluation of the group sessions by participants was requested by the group leaders. Two of the questions the leaders generally asked were: (1) What was most useful and least useful in the group sessions? (2) What should have been discussed that wasn't included?

Conclusions

The group sessions were beneficial for the adjustment of the individual older adults who participated. One such woman had come into the home after having hoped to live her life out in her own home since she was already quite advanced in age. Her husband had been dead for some years, and she had been living independently by herself for some time. She had been an active member of her community and active in business; despite her age, her mind remained alert. She was concerned about those around her, including her neighbors and the local merchants with whom she dealt. Then, as is often the case, she finally acceded to the worries of her family regarding her well-being. They were concerned that she might fall, be in pain but unable to obtain help for herself. Rather than continuing to worry them, she agreed to come into the home. Her agreement did not make the adjustment easier. In the group she talked many times of her home, her garden, neighbors, merchants, etc., that had been or were still in the community. In addition, she had had a pet that was quite aged. She had given this pet to one of her relatives when she gave up her home, but she was quite worried about the pet. She was concerned that its care might not be the same as she might so lovingly furnish. During the sessions this lady was able to talk about her feelings. She gained a good deal of support from the other group members. She discovered that not only did the other group members share and understand her feelings but also that some of their relatives knew each other. The group meetings gained in importance to her as these things were shared. She began to brighten and a wry sense of humor began to be obvious. She began giving as much support to the other group members as she received from them. By the end of the group sessions this lady had not worked through all of her feelings completely but had made a good beginning. She had made close friendships within the group and was visiting those individuals in their rooms between group sessions. These attachments helped fill the void of her losses in coming into the home. The staff of the home also noticed a change in her. It was now easier to get her involved in the activities in the home and have a positive conversation with her.

Those who participated in these groups uniformly expressed a great deal of satisfaction with the sessions. They appreciated that they were asked to participate and that this time was arranged by the staff of the nursing home so that they could meet together with other people who were also involved in this transition process. Workshop participants usually showed some pride in being included in the group. Their roommates and the other residents in the home were often curious about the group. As a result, group members felt special because they were included. Almost always they expressed a great deal of regret that the meetings would end and spent some time exploring ways to continue the friendships begun in the group. In response to this, some of the nursing homes arranged to keep the group members within the home together in various ways. One home scheduled "coffee klatches" for the group members on a regular basis. Another home gave the group members the function of helping other elderly individuals as they came into the home. It is important to note in this regard that the regularly scheduled group endeavors such as activity, recreational, or occupational therapy in nursing homes do not seem to provide the same opportunity to share feelings, etc., which was the basis of this group. The other activities in the home are focused upon more or less specific tasks. While these tasks encourage socialization, they do not provide for a deeper expression of each individual's feelings. The group sessions under discussion here did focus upon the individual.

There were many positive effects of the group noted both by the staffs within the nursing homes where the groups have been scheduled and by the leaders of the group. Among these were an establishment of lasting friendships in addition to a general increase in socialization, improvements in memory, a more optimistic outlook on life, and other improvements in attitudes. The Name Game and the emphasis on finding ways to help to remember did seem to enhance memory among workshop participants. The sharing of solutions to problems in the home and encouragement to try these solutions with the support of the group together with the improvements in memory enhanced self-esteem.

The older adults who come into the nursing home often feel they are at the end of the road. When they find they can improve their memory or that they can still effect changes in their environment, when they find they can retain some independence by solving some of their own problems rather than being totally dependent on others for deciding everything, they experience an increase in self-esteem. No matter how small the task to be accomplished or the improvements made, it seems necessary for people to keep trying, accomplishing something and feeling successful at something. This is an important thought to keep in mind for those who work with the elderly. The group experience discussed above increased self-esteem and facilitated adjustment. Procedures such as these are easy to adapt to nursing home routines. Hopefully, they will gain acceptance so that the difficult adjustment of this transition into a nursing home can be made easier for large groups of elderly.

Recommended Readings

Borup, J. H., Gallego, T. T., and Hefferhan, P. G. *Geriatric relocation,* Ogden, Utah: Weber State College Press, 1978.

Brody, E. M. *A social work guide for long-term care facilities.* Rockville, MD: NIMH, 1974.

Herr, J. J. and Weakland, J. H. *Counseling elders and their families.* New York: Springer, 1979.

Silverstone, B. and Hyman, H. K. *You and your aging parents.* New York: Pantheon Books, 1976.

Tobin, S. S. and Lieberman, M. A. *Last homes for the aged.* San Francisco: Jossey-Bass, 1972.

Part II

Volunteers, Peer Counselors, and Training

7

The Volunteer Connection

Helena C. Hult

A number of studies have highlighted the need of people for human contact and the special benefits of such contact to elderly, confined isolates (For example, see Cohen, 1974; Faulkner, Heisel, and Simms, 1975; Toseland and Sykes, 1977.) These elderly may be struggling against loneliness, against the systems which provide their income, be they public or private, and against dependency upon peers, children, or the very society which seems to negate their humanity and their rights under the law.

Chronic or catastrophic illness may have taken physical as well as financial toll. Cultural conditioning may have robbed them of their ability to seek and find emotional ties when lifelong peers are gone or to seek professional help when needed. Although we are nearing the end of the industrial revolution, according to many economists, the power of the dollar to generate conspicuous consumption remains, somehow diminishing humanity's consciousness of the needs of the poor, the handicapped, and the infirm retired.

With United States population over age 65 predicted to be 31.8 million by the year 2000 (Samuelson, 1978), some innovative planning needs to be done for this large segment of our population.

One fast-growing solution to the problem of human contact for isolated elderly is neighborhood or organizational supporting networks, and in recent years, many agencies have sprung up—the Retired Senior Volunteer Program (RSVP), senior service centers, councils on aging, nutrition programs, day-care and day-activity centers, and health and recreation programs. These in turn have generated other programs with more focused therapeutic potential, such as homemaker services, home health aides, senior companion programs, friendly visiting, or a number of "telephone reassurance" projects. These have been funded largely by government grants under the Older Americans Act and several cooperating federal agencies. However, the funds are seldom sufficient to employ enough highly qualified personnel, which means that an agency often can't make it without volunteers. Hence, the people who hold a well-functioning social service agency together are the volunteers, many of them retired professionals who are increasingly responsive to the needs of their peers. They choose to give their services for limited periods of time in ways that have meaning for them.

One Senior Service Center

For three years the Senior Service Center of the Santa Monica YWCA (since July 1, 1978, the Santa Monica Westside Multiservice Center of the Voluntary Action Center) depended heavily upon its volunteer staff of 50 to 100 people a month. More than one-third of the volunteers were retired professionals: educators, accountants, nurses, social workers, psychologists, writers, dietitians, bankers, administrators of all kinds. The other 64 percent were students, clerical workers, drivers, receptionists, and many others. All of them were absolutely necessary to the delivery of services in information and referral, escort and transportation, legal aid, in-home help, and especially case management, which was necessitated by an increasing number of frail elderly clients who needed multiple services including, for most of them, counseling.

As a former administrator of two agencies for the aging, I believe some of the best therapy is done by first getting to the roots of the emotional crises, which often are not primarily psychological or medical, but rather economic or social, sometimes deriving from legal and bureaucratic confusions and misunderstandings.

Our Senior Service Center was fortunate in having an evaluation team made up of a retired clinical psychologist, a retired associate professor of nursing administration, and a paralegal social worker. Following client assessment, key members of other agencies involved, such as mental health, family services, public social services, etc., were brought into a case-management team, meeting biweekly or as needed to set limits of intervention, goals, objectives, and timelines for meeting needs of mutual clients. The Center staff, which consisted of three full-time and two part-time employees, could not have delivered such necessary service without these highly skilled volunteers, whose worth to the Center was shown by the attitude of gratitude and warmth exhibited by everyone. The volunteer staff was always included in weekly meetings as well as in ad hoc mini-conferences when crises occurred.

Not only because of their expertise, but especially because of their wisdom and experience and their beneficent effects upon frail vintage clients, they were able in a friendly, nonclinical way to counsel when indicated. The volunteers went far beyond assigned hours in their concern. They became the consistent therapeutic support system for the lonely and often disoriented client. They helped secure the public administrator's assistance when evaluation warranted it; they helped families in their dilemmas dealing with elderly relatives; they helped the elderly to move toward protective services when indicated. Public funding or even the considerable private support of the agency could never have afforded such high-priced talent, which was being freely and abundantly given. A case in point will illustrate.

Indirect but Effective Therapy

Case Example

Amelia. When she first came into the Senior Service Center, Amelia was withdrawn, uncommunicative, fearful, and obviously distressed. She picked at her clothes, which hung too loosely on her tall, bony frame. She nervously smoothed her straight gray hair, pulled back from her pale face into a tight bun at her nape. Her huge amber eyes were red-rimmed and almost brimming over.

After a couple of hesitant starts she said, "I have been helping others through the system most of my adult life, and now when I need help, there's no one left to remember, and no one to help me." I asked if she'd like to come into my office. She looked startled and said, "No, no." She had seen too much of offices as her story unfolded, in an almost inaudible voice.

"I was a social worker. I retired several years ago and felt sure I could have a decent retirement. I became very ill, and costs not covered by Medicare ate up my savings, and I have only $256 a month Social Security and I got this three weeks ago from them saying I owe them money!" Her tears spilled over.

She thrust a paper into my hands and told me how she had tried to have the error traced and corrected. She walked miles from office to office because she had no telephone nor the dime for the senior bus fare. Her one-room apartment rent had gone up from $150 to $245 in six months, so that she was surviving on $11 a month for food and everything else.

Just then our volunteer paralegal social worker, Beatrice, entered for her regular three-hour duty. I introduced Amelia to Beatrice, who, in her soft, gentle way, persuaded Amelia to come into her office.

There began an intense labor of caring. Beatrice looked into Amelia's records and discovered she should have been receiving $316 a month for many months and that she had other benefits due her because of her chronic residual illness. Not only did Amelia not owe the government money, but the government owed *her* $3,100 as a result of rulings Amelia didn't know about. Soon the reimbursement check came, due to the paralegal worker's quiet persistence.

She helped Amelia find a much less expensive place to live outside high-rent Santa Monica, so Amelia could afford to pay the first and last month's rent, security deposit, and costs of moving. Even there, the volunteer found movers who did the job for one-third the cost of other movers. The Center's volunteer evaluation team recognized that some of Amelia's aberrant thinking might be due to malnutrition. The volunteers became Amelia's friends, shopped with her, and when she dropped into the Center several months later, we all had a view of what Amelia, who represents the almost 25 percent of persons over age 60 in Santa Monica, must have been like during her career days—though she still was withdrawn. Her gratitude was deeply moving. Shortly after that visit, her son, who lived a distance away, wrote his thanks. His own illness had prevented his helping his mother, and he worried about her.

Commentary. Needless to say, not a great many of the 18,000 requests for assistance received at the Center that year were so dramatically resolved, but in every instance volunteers worked together with staff to ease the despair, assisting in securing just benefits, in finding low-cost in-home help, and in working with doctors, hospitals, and convalescent homes in the clients' best interests. Close linkages with other social services made possible comprehensive care for those no longer able to function well alone or resistive to the available mental health treatment.

The Role of Paraprofessionals

The volunteer drivers of the Senior Service Center also acted as therapeutic support companions. Every one of them formed attachments for particular clients who looked to them for assistance on many things besides transportation: taxes, shopping and consumer complaints, going to social security and other government offices, and more.

Case Examples

Mrs. Werner. One morning the Center received an urgent call from the city. A worried out-of-town daughter of 82-year-old Mrs. Werner had tried to reach her mother by telephone in Santa Monica. She called her every day at that hour, but that day Mrs. Werner did not answer. It happened that Joe, a Senior Service Center driver who knew Mrs. Werner, was in at that moment waiting for his next assignment.

Joe sped to Mrs. Werner's apartment, found her comatose on the bedroom floor, picked her up and brought her to Santa Monica Emergency Hospital. The woman was rushed to surgery, where a team of doctors found a ruptured aortal aneurism and were able to save her.

Joe called the daughter before surgery to say he would meet her if she came to town by plane. She planned, however, to drive, since she lived less than two hours away, but she would be pleased to meet Joe when she arrived.

Mrs. Werner's recovery was rapid. Joe visited her every day, bringing her groceries and the things she needed when she came home from the hospital. He arranged for day-help for her through the Center.

In May, during the Month of the Older American, Mrs. Werner attended the annual open house and party at the Center. At the close of the program, she rose with great dignity and said, "If it were not for you beautiful people I would not be here. If Joe had not been so quick and kind and helpful, I would not have recovered as well as I did. I want everybody to know that. Thank you, and thank God for you."

Commentary. More than 100 clients annually were served in this intensive way, largely by volunteers, both professional and nonprofessional.

Some of the most effective nontraditional therapeutic services to the elderly have come about through the churches. Palisades Presbyterian Church, Pacific Palisades, California, formed an emergency service for those needing help which they called Volunteers in Service Here (FISH). FISH provides emergency supplies, emergency transportation, and money for those who are in temporary dire straits. An example of the kinds of service this group perform follows:

Harry. An older man named Harry called FISH to ask for transportation to the doctor. At that time there was no public or private modified van service that could manage his wheelchair, which he needed because he was severely handicapped from a childhood bout with polio.

The FISH volunteer found a driver with a large enough car to transport the client to the doctor, and a strong friendship ensued between the young driver and the older handicapped man.

This became a long-term caring relationship in which the driver saw that Harry received due benefits which he had not been receiving; that affordable housing was found for him; that suitable companions were employed to assist him with the normal functions of living. In general the young driver became a supportive, kind, and loving friend whom the elder called upon for many needs. This burden became rather heavy, at times, for the volunteer, but he always made the time to help.

Commentary. ACTION has, since 1972, been the independent government arm which funds and monitors national volunteer services such as RSVP and partially subsidized services like the Foster Grandparent Program (FGP) and the Senior Volunteer Program. The latter added a new dimension to American Life—the stipended volunteer—which makes possible the participation of limited-income persons in partially volunteer work.

Studies made of these programs demonstrated the great need of older people for other people who care and have skills to share. Most beneficial seemed to be the restoration of positive self-image, feelings of personal worth, and re-engagement in life of both the elderly who are served and the elderly who serve.

Volunteers Help to Narrow the Generation Gap

Another result of such programs has been a narrowing of the "generation gap." Crossroads School, a private college preparatory school in Santa Monica, worked with the Senior Service Center in an Adopt-a-Grandparent program. Eleventh and twelfth graders in boy–girl teams of two were profiled by the Center's coordinator of volunteers and matched as closely as possible with elderly isolated clients in the Santa Monica Bay Area, who became their "grandparents" for a school year.

Teams visited their grandparents for two or three hours each week, chatting, running errands, taking oral histories, and in many instances acting as advocates for them. One student, Danny, who had a particularly difficult grandparent, got her into a low-cost family practice clinic for competent medical supervision for her many chronic problems and secured nutrition counseling. Highly intelligent and perceptive, Danny concluded that her original doctor was quite intolerant and lacking in understanding of the elderly.

The partnership between school and senior center, between youth and age, has many advantages. It helps to develop and broaden social consciousness on the part of both young and old and adds new dimensions to the school curriculum—in oral history, the arts, journal and script writing, and family skills, for example. It opens up fresh avenues of communication which can lead to personal friendships and widened social understandings.

Many of these features are brought out in a color videotape of one grandparent team, "Thelma and Cindy," developed by the General Telephone Company, which has won wide acclaim. It has become a teaching tool, used by Marian Marshall, director of the California State Department of Adult Education, and by the Leonard Davis School of the Andrus Gerontology Center at the University of Southern California. The videotape has also been featured in several regional workshops on aging.

The Northwest Pilot Project

The formal linking of youth and the elderly isolate actually developed earlier in several areas of the United States. One notable example is the Northwest Pilot Project in Portland, Oregon, which began in 1969, sponsored by Friendly House. The goal of this volunteer service to older people is to enable them to maintain their well-being and dignity within their place of residence. The services offered cover a wide range: information and referral, friendly visiting, escort and transportation, housing, and management services in downtown hotels. Up to 100 volunteers a month work in the project, many of them students.

Case Examples

Mr. Ziegler. A student at Portland State University volunteered to be a friend to Mr. Ziegler, a withdrawn and somewhat difficult old gentleman. Early visits were spent chatting, watching fights on television, drinking coffee, and swapping stories. In the second month of the relationship the volunteer reported:

> Mr. Ziegler seems to trust me. He has been having trouble with his watch. He wants to know if I could help him see that his watch is fixed. Mr. Ziegler is very independent and doesn't like to ask anyone for favors.

A year later, the volunteer reported that Mr. Ziegler's physical condition continued to be weak but stable, although the slightest exercise resulted in shortness of breath. The volunteer continued to stress Mr. Ziegler's desire to remain independent:

> He becomes very upset if he thinks he is the object of anyone's charity . . . but he does seem to trust me, and I have noticed some subtle changes taking place. For example, I might make a suggestion that a certain food item might be better suited to his health needs, and after a few weeks that item may appear on his shelf. But neither of us will say anything about it.

Before long it developed that Mr. Zeigler had multiple medical problems requiring hospitalization. The volunteer helped to provide tender care during his hospital stay and was one of the small group present later at his funeral services.

Karen. The Northwest Pilot Project has also set up a series of summer camps for the elderly who live in downtown Portland hotels. High school volunteers assist with the camp program, often forming lasting one-to-one relationships with their older companions. Youth and staff together involve the campers in activity planning, and some results have been strikingly rehabilitative. For example, some unscheduled participation was shown by Karen, a blind, lame, and withdrawn woman who was present at a stellar production of "My Fair Lady." She got to her feet and began dancing and swinging her cane. When she returned to her hotel, she began taking an active interest in those around her and developed a deep friendship with the youthful volunteer who was her mentor. She even participated in cabin-competition special events. However, when the young volunteer moved away and there was no one to take his place back in the city, the "cane lady" slipped back into apathy and isolation. This emphasizes the importance of a sustained relationship to many older persons; as long as someone cares personally about them, they can remain engaged in the life about them.

Claire. But there are fortunate exceptions. Claire, a 70-year-old woman, had been released from a mental hospital to live in one room in an inner-city Portland hotel. She began to retreat again into her private world. Claire was befriended by a college student volunteer who, after several months of nurturing, established trust so that she shared some of her poetry with the student. The older woman's lifelong love of poetry, both reading and writing it, had never before been shared with anyone. She began to join others in the hotel dining room, and eventually shared her poems with her peers. The love and respect she received in return stimulated her creativity, and for Valentine's Day she wrote a poem for each of the 45 older people who had come to share her life! The volunteer's trust and recognition of her skill so reinforced Claire's selfhood that when her young friend returned to school she continued to accept her responsibility to contribute to the life around her.

Who and Where Are the Volunteers?

We have given examples showing the importance of volunteers in carrying out the various kinds of nontraditional therapy. It may be helpful to conclude with a brief account of the volunteer movement and the major organizations in which volunteers can be found.

Volunteers have been a part of the fabric of human life since the beginning of recorded history. There have always been those persons highly motivated to accept responsibility for the health, education, and welfare of others.

A comparatively recent phenomenon, however, is the recognition of voluntarism in the United States as a significant contribution to the gross national product. In the last decade this force has grown to more than 55,000,000 persons—more than one in four of us—accounting for approximately $35 billion annually in donated time and talent. That figure does not include the billions of dollars raised by volunteers annually in support of causes ranging from the Asthma Foundation to Zero Population Growth.

The formalizing of nonspecific volunteer services began in this country after World War I, when thousands of Red-Cross-trained wartime volunteers returned to peacetime activity. They were eager to put their expertise to work in community service. Hence began offices for volunteer recruitment, referral, and placement, for the most part under auspices of Community Chests (Davis, 1975). Later, these separate volunteer bureaus organized into the Association of Volunteer Bureaus of America which, building upon excellent training and management materials developed by the Red Cross, set standards for performance and accreditation of member bureaus. There are now several professional volunteer societies which monitor and accredit within their specialties.

Important in the development of responsible volunteer programs has been the Association of Junior Leagues, incorporated in 1921 with the stated goal of "education for responsible citizenship through efficient volunteer service." Today there are 236 Junior Leagues in the national association with a membership of more than 127,000, according to the 1978 League handbook.

The Junior League and the Council of Jewish Women (founded in 1883, with a 1978 membership of more than 100,000) often work together, identify needs in a community, carefully plan a method of meeting those needs, including seed money, and then turn over the program to an appropriate agency for maintenance and continued development. For example, the Junior League is now working with the Santa Monica Westside Multiservice Center in the development of one or more activity centers. The purpose is to provide a sheltered, professionally staffed center where elderly parents, isolated live-alones, and the handicapped may come during daytime hours for carefully planned activity, good nutrition and nutrition education, health monitoring, and counseling. The League members not only do preliminary research and costing but pledge their volunteer service for one to five years to assure the solid foundation necessary to win community support for continuing development.

Volunteer organizations in the United States thus provide a reservoir of motivated and public-spirited persons who can be called on to assist with therapeutic programs for older people. With training such as that given to peer counselors, some of them can make a substantial contribution to the morale and mental health of the elderly.

Furthermore, the groundwork has been laid for international cooperation through the International Association for Volunteer Education (IAVE). This organization first met in Los Angeles in 1970 and has had three worldwide conferences on voluntarism, attended by delegates from several dozen nations. Its goals are (1) to remain a nonpolitical influence for peace through sharing health, education, and welfare volunteer experiences which have been helpful and innovative in their own countries for possible adoption elsewhere, and (2) to strengthen bridges of understanding through joining hands and hearts in concerted efforts to further the highest quality health, education, and welfare programs for all people of the world, through skilled volunteer leadership.

The dominant theme throughout correspondence and conferences is creative response to the needs of people from cradle to grave. The present objective of IAVE is to establish an international resource bank of successful volunteer programs around the world so that when a country has a particular need, the bank can supply

Pets Can Be Therapeutic

The Junior League of Boston, Massachusetts, has developed a Pet Therapy Project for the elderly in rest homes. The inspiration behind the Pet Therapy Project originated with a *Boston Globe* story of a lonely elderly gentleman living in a rest home. With no family, friends, or employment, he either rocked in his chair or slept, to avoid the emptiness of a world to which he would no longer relate. One day, a homeless puppy came in from the streets and found the gentleman. The two have grown to love one another, and the gentleman's outlook on life has been immeasurably improved. (*LIVE,* newsletter of the International Association for Volunteer Education, Winter, 1978–79.)

Working with the Massachusetts Society for the Prevention of Cruelty to Animals, the Junior League has begun to place animals in rest homes. Volunteers receive basic training in geriatrics, veterinary care, and animal training.

The goal of the Pet Therapy Project is to enrich the lives of the elderly in rest homes by adding to their sense of purpose and fulfillment through the companionship of animals.

"A pet can provide a boundless measure of love, adoration, and unqualified approval. Many elderly and lonely individuals have discovered that pets satisfy their needs and enable them to hold on to the world of reality, of care," said Dr. Boris Levenson, professor of psychology and author of *Pets and Human Development.*

helpful information and can also put that country in touch with a resource person or persons in a nearby country where the program has been successful.

Third world countries, out of the creative energy of building "a new land," are developing unusual answers to social problems through volunteer effort and leadership. They share with us and we share with them.

The volunteer and the vulnerable elderly have a strong partnership, whether it be in the hills of North Carolina or the mountains of Nepal, the tropical jungles of Brazil or the sun-kissed Isle of Bali. The elderly have much to teach about life and living, about history as it was lived, and about human values.

There are few walls or chasms where love and caring cannot build bridges of communication and sharing.

Recommended Readings

Sainer, J. S. and Sander, M. L. *Serve: older volunteers in community service.* New York: Community Service Society, 1971.

Schindler-Rainman, E. and Lippett, R. *The volunteer community.* Richmond, VA.: United States Learning Resources Corporation, 1971. (Rev. Ed., 1975).

Schindler-Rainman, E., Lippitt, R., Carey, C. M., and Hardy, J. M. *Voluntarism: confrontation and opportunity.* New York: National Council of YMCA's, 1975.

Schindler-Rainman, E., Lippitt, R., and Fox, R. S. *Towards a humane society: images of potentiality.* Ann Arbor, Mich.: NTL Learning Resources Corporation, Inc., 1973.

Spiegel, H. *Concepts and issues: citizen participation in urban development.* Washington, D.C.: Center for Community Affairs, 1968.

U.S. volunteers in action: people helping people. *U.S. News and World Report,* 1971.

8

A Peer Counseling Program in Action

Bernice Bratter and Estelle Tuvman

> I want you to know what Mrs. F. B. did for me. I used to cry a lot and I was so depressed and after my third visit with her I was myself again. She is so kind and understanding and me being a shy person, she made me feel so at ease I just opened up to her.
>
> I want to thank you and Mrs. B. and we are lucky to have people like you to help us.

> I greatly appreciate, much more than this word can express, your time to visit me, and your Sincere Concern, especially, at my time of feeling more and more, the need for that.
>
> Wishing you both also everyone else in your office, the best health possible and the best luck in your excellent work.

In peer counseling, people help each other. The above letters from counselees demonstrate how well the concept is working. Its uniqueness lies in the fact that trained men and women who are not professionals work with persons of similar age and experience. The method has strong appeal for both the helper and the helped. As Hurvitz (1970) concluded, the client responds positively to the peer counselor, and the counselor gains increased self-awareness, self-esteem, and feelings of accomplishment. It is one of the best ways to overcome the resistance shown by older people to professional therapists and counselors. The peer concept facilitates the establishment of a

PEP (Peer Counseling for Elderly Persons) is a program of the Santa Monica Bay Area Health Screening Clinic for the Elderly.

special rapport between two individuals or within a group that allows a genuine supportive relationship to develop.

Since multiple losses and increased depressive reactions are characteristic of old age, the need for mental health services for the elderly is substantial. Yet, as a group, they are inadequately served by mental health professionals.

According to the latest census, 22 percent (20,000) of the population of the city of Santa Monica are over 60 years of age as compared with the national figure of 15 percent. While some mental health services are provided in the Santa Monica and West Los Angeles areas, these programs are crisis oriented rather than preventive.

Medicare rarely reimburses more than three social worker visits after a hospital discharge. Mental health clinics have limited means for responding to the needs of older persons experiencing emotional difficulties. Institutionalization too often becomes the common approach to dealing with their emotional disorders. Butler (1970) has estimated that at least 40 percent of the elderly now institutionalized would not be if there were proper support systems developed to meet their psychosocial needs.

Fortunately, an existing organization, the Santa Monica Bay Area Health Screening Clinic for the Elderly, took action. This nonprofit community agency was formed in 1975 to improve health care services for the elderly in the western part of Los Angeles County. Its emphasis is preventive, and its philosophy focuses on treatment of the total person. Health problems are seen as involving both physical and psychosocial components.

From the beginning, it was clear that many persons seen at the Health Screening Clinic were suffering from depression, anxiety, and loneliness, emotional stresses which were adversely affecting their physical health. Since older people tend to resist professional psychiatric and psychological services, and as there were no other services available in the community to help them, some kind of assistance was necessary. Peer counseling looked like the answer.

Initiating the Program

In view of this situation, the Health Screening Clinic applied to the State Department of Mental Health for a grant to provide a carefully screened group of 25 men and women aged 55 years and older who would be professionally trained and supervised to do peer counseling. A three-year grant was received. The next step was to recruit a training coordinator and a program assistant. This was done through the cooperation with USC's Andrus Gerontology Center and the two leading graduate schools for training social workers.

The first task was to identify 25 mature adults with the potential and commitment to become peer counselors. Plans were made for recruiting, screening, and training.

Recruitment of trainees was done through radio, newspaper, and community newsletter announcements, speaking to local groups, contacting staff at community agencies and centers for the elderly, and distributing letters and flyers. Every effort was made to select a group of counselors who would be representative of the area in which they would serve. Minority leaders in the community were contacted personally. Letters and flyers, sent to all local churches and organizations with high minority involvement, were followed up by a phone call and personal interview whenever possible.

Screening took place in three stages: by (1) telephone; (2) in-depth written application, accompanied by a description of the training and a fact sheet; and (3) personal interviews done in small groups. An evaluation form was developed, based on the essential qualities of the counselor, as suggested in the writings of Leona Tyler (1969), Carl Rogers (1957), and Truax and Carkhuff (1967). Much to the amazement of the staff, more than 200 inquiries were received from potential peer counselors. Sixty-two candidates were interviewed and evaluated jointly by the training coordinator and program assistant. The 25 counselors selected ranged in age from 50 to 82 years and included eighteen women and seven men. Their mean age was 63. Selected peer counselors came from diverse educational, ethnic, and economic backgrounds. They were a multilingual group, speaking Spanish, Yiddish, German, Italian, Polish, and French. A two-year commitment to the program was asked of all the peer counselors, with six hours per week set as the minimum participation. Twenty-four peer counselors remain active with the program, over a year after training was initiated. Stroke and the resultant paralysis and speech impairment changed the role of one of the peer counselors. She maintains contact with the staff and other peer counselors, who provide her with a strong support system. Though she is inactive, everyone still considers her a member of the group.

To maximize the effectiveness of the training program, the training coordinator reviewed the literature related to the counseling of the older adult and the psychosocial aspects of aging. Books purchased and reviewed for the program included: Robert Butler and Myrna Lewis, *Aging and Mental Health* (1977); Robert Butler, *Why*

Survive? Being Old in America (1975); Simone de Beauvoir, *Coming of Age* (1972); Arthur Schwartz, *Survival Handbook for Children of Aging Parents* (1977). Numerous journal articles were reviewed and duplicated to develop a resource library for the peer counselors.

The training coordinator, the program assistant, and the project director met with staff members of the USC Andrus Gerontology Center who were directly involved with the actual design, writing, and implementation of the Peer Counseling program and training manual.

A two-part training program, using *Counseling the Older Adult* (Alpaugh and Haney, 1978) as the text, was designed. Two months of classes, meeting twice weekly for three hours per session, were scheduled. The Santa Monica Department of Parks and Recreation provided a site for the training. Co-trainers (from USC's Andrus Gerontology Center) experienced in peer counseling led the first month of the training, which began with an orientation and "get-acquainted" session. A class roster and list of available reading materials were distributed.

The purpose of the curriculum was to (1) enhance personal qualities essential in good counselors—empathy, respect, genuineness; (2) increase self-awareness through the counselor's own self-development; (3) develop the counseling skills of active listening and problem-solving; (4) familiarize the counselors with facts about aging that are essential in the counseling of older adults; (5) acquaint counselors with community resources. The sessions for both the first and second months involved lectures, group discussions, and small group exercises designed to practice counseling skills.

During the second month of training, professionals working with the elderly volunteered to do workshops on (1) group process, (2) government resources—social security, Medicare, Medi-Cal, (3) cross-cultural counseling, (4) human sexuality, (5) depression, grief, anxiety, (6) crisis intervention and suicide, (7) stress reduction and relaxation, (8) community resources and referrals, and (9) record-keeping.

Throughout the training period, the training coordinator held individual conferences with the trainees to assess their response to the program and analyze their individual needs during the course.

Certificates for completion of training were awarded at a graduation ceremony. The new peer counselors shared their sense of achievement with friends, relatives, and staff members of community agencies who were invited to attend.

After their formal training, trainees needed practice in counseling techniques as well as more information about the population they would serve. Many were anxious about their ability to be effective counselors.

To provide both support and further experience, the peer counselors were divided into two groups for two-and-a-half hours of weekly supervision. The supervision is a continuing program in which cases are reviewed and role playing used for practicing counseling skills. Among the programs conducted are assertiveness training, management of depression, death and dying, evaluation of institutional care, working with the disabled, and life review as a technique for counseling. Also, the peer counselors are informed of community programs which would enhance their knowledge or skills. Ongoing training and supervision have served to maintain a high level of interest on the part of the peer counselors as well as to improve their counseling effectiveness and self-confidence. The training coordinator and the program assistant continue to be available to the peer counselors for individual supervision whenever needed.

Introducing the Peer Counseling Program to the Community

To introduce the peer counseling program, a variety of approaches were utilized. The training coordinator, the project director, and the program assistant contacted community agencies, clinics, hospitals, and organizations serving the elderly. First a descriptive letter was sent. Phone calls and personal interviews followed. PEP staff spoke to staff of potential referral agencies. A one-page leaflet was distributed widely (see Fig. 1).

The news media have been used to publicize the program by means of radio interviews and public service announcements on various local stations; a television interview on CBS News; newspaper articles in the *Santa Monica Outlook, Los Angeles Times, Independent,* and community newsletters.

In order to reach those persons who would not identify themselves as needing counseling, six rap groups were established at different sites in the community. These groups meet weekly at three nutrition sites, a Senior Recreation Center, a community bank, and a private home.

Peer counselors have appeared before community groups such as RSVP, General Telephone, and the Santa Monica Bay Area Women's Club, presenting educational programs about aging and retirement. They have also presented training programs that focus on the

Figure 1.

SANTA MONICA BAY AREA
HEALTH SCREENING CLINIC FOR THE ELDERLY, INC.
1148 4th St. Santa Monica, Calif. 90403
394-8611

pep

PEER COUNSELING FOR ELDERLY PERSONS

BOARD OF DIRECTORS

GOLDA LARKS
President
JAMES FREED, D.D.S.
Vice President
BEATRICE MISHKIN
Secretary
DAN SULLIVAN
Treasurer

GERALD SHAW, M.D.
FRANCES COHEN, R.N.
RUTH MILLS
LOUISE GABRIEL
NATHAN MATLIN
CYNTHIA DIERKES
CORA KLEINER
RALPH SACHS, M.D.
JOHANNE HANSER, R.N.

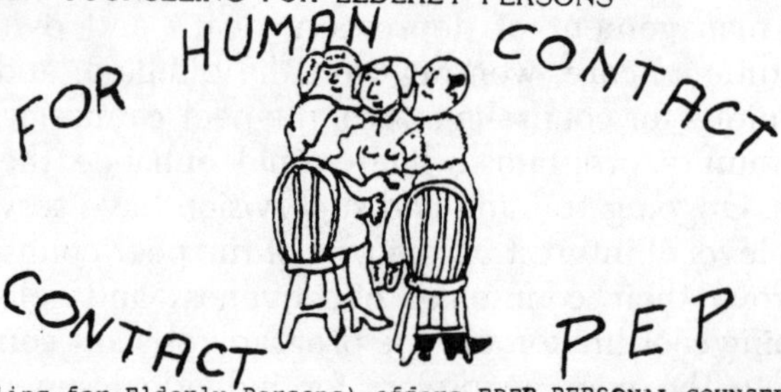

FOR HUMAN CONTACT

CONTACT PEP

PEP (Peer Counseling for Elderly Persons) offers FREE PERSONAL COUNSELING for older adults residing in the greater Santa Monica, Venice and West Los Angeles areas. Counseling is being provided by paraprofessionals aged 55 years and older who have participated in an extensive training program given jointly with USC School of Gerontology. Our counselors are men and women chosen for their warmth, sensitivity, compassion and broad life experiences. They receive ongoing professional supervision and continuing education.

It is our objective to assist the older person to remain in the community enjoying a greater sense of independence and self-esteem. With Peer Counseling, older adults can experience a supportive relationship with someone their own age which leads to a renewed sense of involvement and well-being.

PEP is sponsored by the Santa Monica Health Screening Clinic for the Elderly and is funded by the California State Department of Health. Our counselors are available at the clinic, selected community agencies and for home visits.

For further information call 394-8611.

Bernice Bratter
Coordinator

Judy Gewertz
Program Assistant

development of communication and counseling skills for participants working with the elderly in such programs as Volunteers for Victim Assistance and Crime Prevention, Nursing Home Advocates, and cab drivers and phone operators with Yellow Cab's Dial-a-Ride. This diversified utilization of peer counselors expands the general concepts of the program and greatly increases its outreach potential. In addition, such involvement has contributed positively to the growth and development of the peer counselors.

Sources of referrals have been the Health Screening Clinic, nutrition sites, Santa Monica Hospital, Brotman Memorial Hospital, St. John's Hospital, Kaiser-Permanente Hospital, Visiting Nurses Association, RSVP, Santa Monica Emeritus College, Senior Service Center, Senior Recreation Center, Didi Hirsch Community Mental Health Center, St. Ann's Church, Family Service of Santa Monica, Adat Shalom Temple, private physicians, Home Health Services, personal referrals, and self-referrals.

The demand for peer counselors to do counseling, act as group facilitators, and do community programs has far exceeded the original expectations of the program. In the first four months of taking referrals, more than twice the number of clients originally set as a three-year program objective were seen.

The latest count, which covers 16 months of referrals from June 1978 through September 1979, shows that we have provided services to 249 persons on an individual basis and have had an attendance of 3,574 persons in rap groups and continuing education programs.

Implementing the Program

The appropriateness of each referral to PEP is evaluated by the professional staff before an individual is accepted into the program. The person's needs, the seriousness of the problem to all concerned, and motivation to be helped are considered. Before a peer counselor is assigned to a case, the training coordinator or program assistant consults with each counselee. This step was initiated after several cases were referred without the consent of the counselees. The majority of counselees are suffering from depression, loneliness, and anxiety.

When a peer counselor is assigned, the counselee is called for the purposes of introduction and setting up of an appointment. Clients meet with counselors on a one-to-one basis or in groups. The majority

Peer Help for the Homebound

Since over 50 percent of the PEP clients are homebound, many individual sessions are held in clients' homes. The initial home visit is supervised by Judy Gewertz, R.N., B.A., the Program Assistant, who cites the following case:

Shirley, a 78-year-old retired schoolteacher, was referred to PEP by a social worker at the hospital where she had undergone rather extensive vascular surgery. When the peer counselors first visited her, she was getting around in her robe and slippers.

She talked to them about her poor health and her need for household help and transportation to the doctor's office. As the hour went on, she began to express her feelings. She was *lonely.* Childless, with no relatives nearby, she had been widowed ten years before when her husband had a massive heart attack and died "sitting right there watching TV!" She was *worried* and *depressed* and seemed unable to make important decisions. The burden of cooking, caring for her home, and managing her finances was too much for her. And she was *angry!* "Sure, he's gone, and I'm left with all these problems!" She needed someone on whom she could rely for warm, caring support. The counselors listened sympathetically, suggested she call the Senior Service Center for transportation and household help and promised to return the following week.

As Shirley grew stronger, she was able to do more for herself and to drive her car. The peer counselors suggested she contact friends, which she did. They helped her work through the problems of managing her finances, including a search for someone to share her house. They enabled her to ventilate anger at her deceased husband. As her depression lessened, she began to cope better with her other problems.

However, the unexpected happened. Shirley fractured her hip and had to be hospitalized. Her peer counselors continued to work with her, helping her explore options for her future living arrangements. She was able to find a pleasant and comfortable guest house, where she is now living. She sold her home, kept her car, and when she was seen last, was happy, content, and able to deal with her problems in a positive and productive way.

of individual counseling sessions are done on a weekly basis for approximately one hour. Groups generally meet for one-and-a-half to two hours on a weekly basis.

A file is kept for each individual client and each rap group. In the rap groups, members sign in for each session. Peer Counselor facilitators (working in pairs) summarize the events of each group meeting for the files. These records are reviewed regularly by the training coordinator and program assistant as an additional means of supervision. Referral agencies are contacted to report the status of clients referred.

Individuals are seen at the Health Screening Clinic, at various sites in the community, and in their own homes. The training coordinator or the program assistant accompanies the peer counselors on each initial home visit for purposes of screening and supervision. Once rapport is established between counselor and client, telephone contact is often maintained between sessions.

During the first phase of the program, all peer counselors worked in pairs. After nine months of training and experience, most of them have been able to work alone and make home visits without a supervisor.

Cases Examples

The day-to-day operation of the program can be seen best by reviewing a few respresentative cases. Peer counselors report the cases of Wanda and Sally.

Wanda. Wanda, 60 years old, was widowed two years ago. Her health is rather poor—she has high blood pressure, angina, and periodic episodes of phlebitis. She has two married daughters, Nancy and Marie. Nancy has two children, a boy and a girl; Marie has one little girl.

We have met fourteen times over a period of five months. Her presenting problem involved her distress over her relationship with her younger sister Martha. They had a long history of arguments in which Martha put her down, accused her of being foolish or stupid, and criticized her endlessly for things she said or did, no matter how trivial. In addition, Martha frequently taunted her with "Mama loved you better than she did me." (Their mother had died many years ago.) Wanda's way of dealing with her sister was always the same—defending and denial; and the results were always the same: she was left feeling frustrated, misunderstood, unjustly accused, anxious, and filled with unexpressed anger. Despite these continually recurring episodes, she loved Martha and worried about presenting her in a bad light to the counselor. The situation was brought to a head for Wanda when she suffered an angina attack after a particularly upsetting incident with Martha. While in the hospital, she was told about PEP by a staff social worker. Up to that time she had read a great many self-help books hoping she could, through them, find a way to improve their relationship, but that didn't happen. While she was recuperating, she decided to come to PEP for help.

She has a good relationship with each of her daughters and told them of her decision. Both had been greatly concerned about her inability to deal effectively with Martha and were very supportive of her decision to get help. However, Wanda was very careful to keep her association with PEP from Martha and her brother and his wife (with whom she has a very good relationship).

During her first session, after describing how she felt after an exchange with Martha, she said, "I know I can't change her, so I'm going to have to change myself, otherwise this situation could kill me."

As counseling continued, Wanda achieved much insight into many aspects of herself. Most pertinent to her presenting problem was the realization that she accepted her sister's evaluations of her actions and behavior as the standards by which she judged herself. This was followed by the recognition that she has the right to set her own standards for herself. She then began to be more assertive and has found, much to her surprise, that Martha has become much less critical.

When she became more comfortable with her assertiveness, Wanda no longer felt it necessary to conceal the fact from Martha that she was getting help and found it quite easy to tell her. She realized that it no longer mattered to her what Martha might think or what her brother and his wife might think and she told them so.

Wanda's change has helped produce change in the others. Her relationship with Martha is no longer a problem to Wanda. As counseling continues, she learns new ways of dealing with other people.

Sally. Sally, a 70-year-old depressed woman, had a very low image of herself, an image she has carried with her since she was a child in a mining town. Busy with the responsibility of looking after several brothers and sisters, she never paid attention to her appearance. Occasionally, she would look into a very small mirror that was hanging on the kitchen wall. When she did, her mother would yell, "Stop looking at yourself—you're just an ugly little thing!" This is how she still perceived herself at age 70.

Actually, Sally has a lively face, beautiful, unwrinkled skin, peaches-and-cream complexion, and light blue eyes. She confessed that she hardly ever looked into a mirror because all she would see was an ugly woman. The counselor encouraged her to see the face in the mirror that others saw—the beautiful face with the lovely eyes and goodness emanating from it. After two months of sessions, she came in one day with a permanent, makeup, and a big smile. Her pleasure with herself was so evident that her counselor grabbed her and hugged her.

This same client revealed that in all of her 70 years she had never eaten in a restaurant, because when she was young her mother had often told her never to eat anywhere but at home. This was the pattern she followed, even after her marriage. She would accompany her husband to a restaurant; he would eat and she would just sit and join him for coffee. He had begged her for years to eat along with him, but her fear of dirt, germs, sickness, etc., was so pronounced that it prevented her from ever eating out. The counselor pointed out to her the exacting health standards and the sanitary conditions that prevail today, which seemed to make some impression. Then the counselor gave her an assignment: to go and eat a meal in a certain restaurant often patronized by the counselor, and guaranteed, by her, to be clean, with wholesome, healthy food.

Lo and behold! The following week Sally came in with a big grin on her face. She had eaten out and had liked it! Asked what her feelings were when she went into the restaurant, she said she was extremely nervous, but she remembered the counselor's words while she was making her choice of foods, and while eating, she heard the same voice telling her "It's safe, Sally. Eat it and enjoy it." So she overcame that hurdle and now both she and her husband are happier and grateful because, for the first time, they can go out and enjoy a meal together.

A definite challenge to the peer counselor is shown in this case of an elderly, bedridden man recuperating from radical surgery. The test came when the patient undressed and the counselor saw how extensive the surgery had been. A first-person report, covering about 22 sessions over a six-month period, is given by the counselor.

Tom. Tom was 83; he came back to his trailer from the hospital after what he thought was a hernia repair. He was totally incontinent, his buttocks lying on a circular air-cushion. He was wearing diapers, which he had to change every two to four hours; his legs were swollen and a fiery red and the peeling wounds on his legs itched uncontrollably. He had breathing difficulties and had an oxygen tank which he used intermittently; he produced great amounts of phlegm, which he expectorated into a metal cup kept close to his couch. He also had high blood pressure. For each of his diseases he had some pills—altogether a tray full—which he took on various schedules. These schedules he had written up on slips of stout paper, but I never understood how he could keep these schedules straight.

It was quite easy to get the medical history, but could I establish immediate contact which would permit at least temporary relief? I noticed little picture-postcards of saints sitting next to his bed. So I began to talk about his religion, whereupon he requested that his priest come every other Sunday, after church, to give him communion at regular intervals. This was my first bridge to Tom. From the beginning of the first session, I was quite overwhelmed with his suffering, which he endured so stoically.

After that, I saw Tom every week. I tried to help him keep up his trailer and his personal laundry, and checked to see that people did the marketing for him. His diet was atrocious, but I didn't criticize it, nor did I comment on his smoking next to the oxygen tank. He felt he could take care of himself and was dead set against a nursing home or hospitalization. We talked about his former life—four marriages, a daughter from one, a son from another. (Both helped within their means.) Telling me about his various jobs (for example, shipyard repair after Pearl Harbor in World War II) provided an opportunity to strengthen his ego and divert attention from his misery. Another vehicle of conversation was his Catholicism, particularly the death of the Pope, the coronation of the next one, his death, and the election of a successor. He wouldn't believe me when I told him that the new Pope was not an Italian. ("The Pope is always an Italian!")—probably because he himself was of Italian descent. But he knew so little of Italy this was not much of a bridge.

On an extremely hot summer day, a neighbor in the trailer court suggested that we drive to the ocean to cool off. For this he had to dress in my presence and I saw the extent of the surgical repair: the whole pelvic region was replaced by a sack-like structure, probably the stretched-out scrotum. No penis was present and instead there was (approximately at the location where one would expect the penis) a small, blood-red circular opening through which urine dribbled. I was deeply shocked at this mutilation (life-saving though it undoubtedly was), and it took a conference with my supervisor and sheer will power for me to stand this sight on subsequent occasions. Looking back, I noted that after this first experience, Tom was no longer hesitant to uncover himself.

Was this the greatest confidence, showing me his mutilated body—his inside, as it were? At any rate, we had a good time through the summer and into the fall. We planned for the future, relived old experiences, and took life from week to week. He had been a strong person who enjoyed life—gambler that he was—in varied situations. He had a gun next to his couch, for self-protection. But his physical condition deteriorated progressively. One day in November, a neighbor in the trailer court called me to report that Tom had taken a turn for the worse. I drove over immediately. Tom was talking of death for the first time. I called his daughter, who took him to Santa Monica Hospital the next day. Shortly thereafter, Sister Wilma from St. Anne's Parish informed me that Tom had died.

"Rap" Groups

The peer counselors worked to set up rap groups for older people in the community. At these meetings problems could be discussed or, at the very least, the seniors could learn about the peer counseling program and ask for individual appointments. At first the counselors found it difficult to get seniors to join groups or, if they did attend, to listen and participate. Turnover was considerable as people explored and tried out the various groups.

After a good deal of promoting, one counselor was delighted when thirteen attended the first meeting, which she thought went quite well and got the group off to a good start. The next week only four returned! She managed to keep the group going but encountered other frustrations. For example, just when one member seemed to be getting insight into an identity problem, and another into a family relationship, both individuals left the group as if fearful of pursuing the matter any further.

The seniors who were interested gravitated into groups which differed greatly. The focus of one group was life reviews given by each member. Another seemed to favor a more superficial involvement with daily events and generally steered clear of feelings. A third group fluctuated between personal problems and the strains of daily living. In contrast, a women's group, meeting in a private home, delved right into each member's emotional problems and established a strongly supportive atmosphere. Their eight to ten members attended consistently one day a week, from 10:30 A.M. to 3:00 P.M., and ate lunch together.

At the time of this writing six groups are alive and functioning, which testifies to the value of the group approach for older people with problems. The following case is a good illustration.

Case Example

Mrs. May. Mrs. May, in her middle to late 60s, began group sessions in September. A slender, neatly dressed, well-groomed woman, she attended faithfully, but always remained very quiet and seldom participated in group discussions. Her discomfort with speaking to the group was apparent, since she would express herself only privately to the group facilitator after the day's discussion.

As the holidays approached in December, the group's discussion turned to reminiscences about childhood. Group members were sharing very positive kinds of experiences as they were remembered. Quite unexpectedly, Mrs. May spoke up in a rather angry voice saying, "I can't find anything delightful in my early memories." At this point the group facilitator turned to Mrs. May and asked her if she would like to share some of her experiences with the group. With great difficulty and emotion—lips quivering and eyes filled with tears—Mrs. May began to unfold her childhood experiences. She described a very unhappy, lonely childhood in which her father deserted the family, after which her mother, out of desperation, placed her four children in an orphanage. Mrs. May was four years old at the time. Her mother removed her from the orphanage when she saw that the child was devastated by the experience. Though she remained with her mother, Mrs. May grew up under circumstances of tremendous poverty and loneliness.

Everyone in the group listened attentively to Mrs. May's life history. They were surprised to find that this very quiet woman had experienced such hardship. The entire group was extremely supportive, and Mrs. May could be seen to relax as she responded to the warmth and support surrounding her.

By revealing herself, Mrs. May took a risk which resulted in her becoming an established member of the group. She discussed her problems more openly during group sessions and no longer needed to speak to the facilitator alone after the group meetings.

A Few Concluding Thoughts

Because our program is new and is still being evaluated in all its phases, it is not yet possible to present many statistics. A few overall figures are of interest, however: Although our original objective was to reach between 200 and 300 counselees within three years, more than five times that number have received our services within the first eight months of full activity.

The data analysis thus far demonstrates that the group being seen is a highly depressed, anxious, lonely older population, predominantly low income and in poor health. A major strength of our program is our affiliation with the Health Screening Clinic. Through cross-referral, we are able to identify and respond to both the physical and emotional needs of our counselees. Although it is too early to have complete pre- and post-test figures on progress made, we have tabulated the first few dozen ratings of peer counselors doing individual and group counseling. Results show that contact with peer counselors is perceived by over 90 percent of the counselees as being either "extremely helpful" or "very helpful."

The data also show that the peer counselors rate the various components of their training as overwhelmingly positive. They themselves were rated by their trainers as quite excellent for beginning counselors. All peer counselors have reported improved self-esteem, self-confidence, and life satisfaction. Their high morale and sense of community is shown by the fact, as already mentioned, that every one of them has remained as a volunteer in the program.*

Recommended Readings

Alpaugh, P. and Haney, M. *Counseling the older adult—a training manual.* Los Angeles: University of Southern California, 1978.

Brammer, L. M. *The helping relationship.* New York: Prentice-Hall, 1973.

Butler, R. N. and Lewis, M. I. *Aging and mental health; positive psychosocial approaches.* St. Louis: C. V. Mosby, 2nd ed., 1977.

Truax, C. and Carkhuff, R. *Toward effective counseling and psychotherapy: training and practice.* Chicago: Aldine, 1967.

Tyler, L. *The work of the counselor.* New York: Appleton-Century-Crofts, 3rd ed., 1969.

*List of Peer Counselors (many of whom assisted in preparing the chapter): Maria Alatorre, Mildred Altfeld, Florence Beer, Leon G. Bennett, Sol P. Blum, Edith Bond, Dorthy Cannaday, August P. DiMille, Evelyn K. Engreen, Fred E. Engreen, Kathleen H. Freeman, Maude I. Haas, Rosemarie Harris, Maudry Mae Harrison, Joseph Heiferman, Sylvia Karp, Varsen Katsky, Blanche Lasher, Michelle A. Macdonald, Minnie H. Meyer, Jan L. Phillips, Jane B. Sinn, Fred S. Topik, Carlos Vega, Eva L. Weiner.

9

Training of Peer Counselors

Arthur N. Schwartz

The purpose of this chapter is to describe the training of nontraditional counselors identified as peer counselors of older people. Simple and straightforward as this task may seem, it has certain pitfalls. One cannot assume, for example, a general consensus in the field about the role of peer counseling (or of nontraditional therapy) or even about the nature of training considered necessary or desirable. We have observed that training in academic settings is likely to follow criteria that provide the best fit with academic training models. These criteria may be at variance with training done in agency contexts or training done under the auspices of religious organizations.

These large variations in assumptions and expectations about the validity, utility, and nature of peer counseling characterize a field of endeavor which is strewn with theoretical and operational landmines. It is certainly not my intent to focus in this chapter on a polemic supporting the validity or utility of peer counseling of older persons, although my case is built on this premise. Such arguments have already been cogently stated (see Schlossberg, 1976; Harrison and Entine, 1976; Troll and Nowak, 1976; Bocknek, 1976). Suffice it to note at this point that the counseling of any age group by their peers is not, in itself, a novel notion. I recall that over a dozen years ago a program was developed on the East Coast (see Reiff and Riessman, 1965) which argued well for the use of peers. It was found that one could capitalize on the street "savvy," the "moxie," and the cultural knowledgeability of the indigenous nonprofessionals (i.e., the neighborhood workers) to provide a counseling type of intervention that produced helpful, even "therapeutic" outcomes. Rioch (1966) has demonstrated the point by training housewives to become competent therapists. What is true of such help offered to younger persons is no less applicable to persons in the later years of life. Indeed, from time immemorial, an important and intrinsic component of the so-called informal support system of elderly people has been the informal counseling response of one elderly person to another when experiencing distress or difficulties.

Given the truly remarkable growth of that "mental health" specialty called therapy—which parallels the pervasive influence of Freudian psychology in the twentieth century—informal, nontraditional counseling by peers continues to exist as a viable, alternative option for those aged who need and seek help by way of talking things over with another concerned, sympathetic human being. Unfortunately, some members of the professional and legal communities look down on peer counseling as of a lesser order than therapy, though the distinction is difficult to maintain operationally. Furthermore, it is implied that the problems dealt with by peer counselors are neither as extensive, as profound, nor as complex as those ordinarily dealt with by professional therapists.

Effects of the Freudian Influence

It is not too difficult to identify some of the reasons which account for such a view. For one thing, orthodox Freudian doctrine has long held the notion that basic personality characteristics are developed and set at a very early stage of development, well within the first decade of life. These basic characteristics, so this view goes, are little, if at all, amenable to modification. Consistent with this, then, is the conclusion that with advanced age the point of no return (with respect to behavioral or personality change) has long since been passed. Given Freud's extreme pessimism about personality or cognitive flexibility in the later years, those who subscribed to his formulations have in the past seen little, if any, payoff to be expected via therapy or analysis for the aged. No doubt this largely accounts for the dismal track record of Freudian psychiatry and psychology with respect to services offered to the elderly. This is evidenced by the fact that training and practice in those disciplines has almost exclusively focused on the young and the middle-aged. At the same time the emotional distress, problems, difficulties, and maladaptations of the elderly have been viewed as merely symptomatic of the expected pathologies intrinsic to old age.

Another reason for the relative disinterest of traditional, professional therapists with respect to old people is the widely held notion that therapy/counseling which merits labels such as "substantive" and "rigorous" invariably requires highly sophisticated techniques and skills, usually involving complex procedures. If emotional disequilibrium and behavioral anomalies in the old are perceived as eruptions (read "symptoms") of severe pathologies of old age, then it would indeed follow that it would take the most skilled technicians utilizing the most sophisticated bag of tricks (along with drugs) to treat and cure the "mentally ill" old. Given the insufficient number of such highly trained and skilled practitioners and their limited time and energy, it is no wonder that cries for help by large numbers of elderly in emotional distress or crisis have been largely ignored or avoided in the name of lack of available manpower. This argument continues to surface periodically even now.

These assumptions and beliefs have led, until very recently, to the conclusion by many practitioners and policymakers that "serious" psychotherapy (usually connoting ongoing, long-term, insight-producing, personality-restructuring intervention) is contraindicated for the aged. Some professionals (reflected in public attitudes) continue to believe that counseling the elderly has no long-range utility. Counseling the old is thus characterized as, at best, superficial stop-gap advice-giving, providing kindly reassurance.

The Need for Peer Counseling

For these reasons, then, counseling the old as a serious, substantial, therapeutic enterprise has fallen outside the framework of the traditional therapeutic domain (Kastenbaum, 1964). Therefore, the growing current interest in training peer counselors to work with older adults and their families has come to be viewed as an interesting and useful adjunct to traditional therapeutic interventions. My own perspective, shared with the editor and contributors to this volume, is that such nontraditional counseling of the elderly is not only a useful but an essential element in the overall configuration of vital services to older adults. In due time, I believe, we shall see such nontraditional counseling become part and parcel of the mainstream of traditional therapies available to the aged.

Even now we can detect emerging trends which demonstrate the effectiveness of training older persons to be counselors of their age peers. Skills training of peer counselors is beginning to take a variety of directions: counseling of marital and sexual problems of the aged, counseling for personal emotional stress, intergenerational conflicts, second and third career options, and for economic, housing, and disability crises, and the like.

The proliferation of peer counselor training and activity obviously is not happening in a vacuum. It reflects and is responsive to a clear and urgent need for such help on the part of graying Americans. It is a phenomenon which also mirrors a growing interest among older persons themselves, regardless of prior occupation or experience, in this kind of helping activity. By the same token, the growth of peer counseling reflects the inadequacy of the mental health community for providing extensive contacts, coverage, and interventions which our elderly appear to require.

In order to understand the context in which peer counseling is growing, two facts need to be set in juxtaposition. One is the well-documented, recognized fact that over 85 percent of the social support enjoyed by America's aged derives from family systems and other neighbor/friendship networks. The second observation is the growing concern of the professional communities, particularly the "mental health" community, over what is described as the underutilization of mental health services and facilities by the aged. Whatever the real reasons may be, it is fair to say that the present cohort of elderly in our society are not turning en masse to those professionals identified and designated as mental health service providers.

It would appear on the surface, at least, that the key to providing grass-roots counseling for needy but reluctant elderly which will reach between the cracks is to be found in training peer counselors who have the prerequisite characteristics to enable them to be effective counselors. Once mental health professionals come to recognize that they (the professionals) can, and should, play a significant role in producing adequate numbers of such nontraditional counselors of the elderly, that their own roles, status, and income are not going to be jeopardized by so doing, we shall see at hand a firm basis for building an efficient, effective, and congenial collaboration between traditional and nontraditional counselors of the elderly (Carp, 1974).

The Process of Selecting Peer Counselors

When it comes to selecting older people who will prove to be effective peer counselors, the state of the art is best described as primitive. Would-be counselors usually come to attention simply because they volunteer for such activity. Motivation and attitudes vary considerably among volunteers, although commonly such persons volunteer because they want to help.

A strong argument for selecting nonprofessional, nondegree peer counselors has been made by Thomas Oden (1974). This point of view insists that the essence of *effective* counseling (that which is most therapeutic) lies not in "tricks of the trade" so much as in certain necessary personality characteristics of the counselor, such as empathy and warmth.

We must acknowledge, therefore, that willingness and good intentions are necessary but not sufficient criteria for selecting potential peer counselors. An older volunteer may want to help others as a counselor, but may see the task merely as well-intentioned (commonsense) advice-giving. Giving advice has its place on occasion, but more often than not when counseling is required, the mere giving of advice may prove to be most disadvantageous, if not disastrous.

Following the formulations of Truax and Carkhuff (1967), the selection of candidates for peer counselor must take into account at least four personal characteristics:

Being a good listener. Good listening skills, as used here, are the sine qua non among those necessary characteristics required of an effective counselor of older adults. Good listening goes beyond a merely passive function. It may be operationally defined as actively attending to what the client is attempting, both verbally and nonverbally, to communicate. It involves the hard work of attempting to comprehend and identify the communication at several levels of understanding.

Hearing and understanding spoken words are intrinsic to effective listening skills, of course. In addition, the good listener must be able to understand (get in touch with, as some put it) what often is not—sometimes cannot be—put into words. The frequently "hidden" message is the feeling tone, the affect, conveyed by nuances in demeanor, tone of voice and inflection, expressiveness or lack of it, body posture, loudness or softness of voice, rate of speech, and what is omitted from the communication, appropriately or inappropriately. Such aspects of the communicative process are subtle, but nevertheless comprise essential dimensions of communication. They are basic to good listening skills as far as counseling is concerned.

Exhibiting accurate empathy. Empathic skill is the ability to put oneself accurately in another's place or circumstance. This is also related to listening skills. A pilot study conducted by the writer and one of his students some years ago illustrates the point.

Veterans seeking admission to a large VA domiciliary were interviewed individually prior to and following each interview the veteran had with information-seeking professionals on the VA staff: admitting physician, ward physician, psychologist, social worker, etc. Following each interview the staff member was asked, "What were the veteran's primary concerns as you understand them? What was he trying to tell you?" In turn, following each interview, the veteran was asked, "What concern were you trying to get across to the staff interviewer?" The veteran was also asked, "Do you think you were understood?" The disparity between what the staff members stated they understood the client to be saying and what the client said he was trying to communicate was, in the majority of instances in this pilot study, quite remarkable. The quality of empathy on the part of the interviewers, as perceived by the interviewees, was often absent. The most frequently stated response of interviewees to the question was, "They didn't seem to understand what I was trying to say."

Unconditional warmth. Over the years, followers of Carl Rogers have called this "nonpossessive warmth." It refers to that quality in a counselor which enables him to accept another as a human being without attaching a "price tag" of one kind or another. Warmth as a personal characteristic does not necessarily imply unconditional agreement with the other person. It is a quality of behavior, however, which does communicate the spirit and feeling of liking the other and emotional (as well as intellectual) responsiveness to the other.

Genuineness. Another important characteristic is genuineness, which means straightforwardness, the ability to share openly in an honest, direct fashion. It translates into self-disclosure when indicated and appropriate to do so. To put it another way, genuineness calls for dealing off the top of the deck with a client, gently but firmly delineating the boundaries of reality insofar as that can be determined, in a consistent, predictable manner. This characteristic of genuineness in a counselor as much as anything else provides the basis for establishing a trusting relationship.

Once the appropriate motivation has been ascertained, these characteristics can and should become criteria for selection of peer counselors. They are necessary but not sufficient predictors of success at counseling older adults. Other additional factors such as reliability, persistence, and ethical integrity will also be involved in determining whether or not the nontraditional counselor will be effective and successful. All these elements can be assessed during the course of training.

Case Example

The following brief case description and commentary will indicate how the personal characteristics described in the foregoing facilitate establishing a working, therapeutic relationship with older clients. It will also indicate how these characteristics manifest themselves as intrinsic, interrelated, interacting aspects of a counselor's responses to an elderly client. These qualities should never be viewed as techniques, moods, attitudinal sets, or tricks of the trade which can be mechanically inserted into the counseling process to achieve a certain effect. In a very real sense the effectiveness of counseling, at least in those many instances where a good relationship is critical, depends most of all upon the kind of person the counselor is.

Mrs. Schmidlap. A 71-year-old widow, Mrs. Schmidlap, came by appointment to see the counselor. Her movements appeared phlegmatic, her speech was mostly halting and slow-paced, her face was anxious, her eyes were sad, her shoulders drooped, and her hands and fingers moved constantly in nervous, at times agitated, fashion. She described episodes of insomnia, recurring headaches, and poor appetite. She appeared distracted and preoccupied. Finally she got to the point. She had been seeing her physician over the past months about increasing visual difficulties. On his recommendation she consulted an ophthalmologist. Following his examination she was told that her prospects were grim; she was facing a 75 percent chance of losing her vision totally. Her son had urged her to get a second opinion, which she did, only to have her worst fears confirmed. Now, again at the urging of her son, she was seeing a counselor for help.

As she, with great reluctance, spilled out her deep-rooted feelings of terror at the thought of going blind and becoming utterly helpless, the counselor began herself to respond with anxiety. While Mrs. Schmidlap was tearfully describing how hopeless and distraught she felt, the counselor became acutely aware of her own sense of frustration and helplessness toward this client. What could she say to reassure or to help? What magic words would calm the panic and stem the flood of tears?

Commentary. Responding with inappropriate reassurance ("it's not as bad as it seems" or "things will work out") can be worse than no response at all because it implies that the client is overreacting to her fears and pain. Rather, the counselor, if an empathic and warm person, will be reassuring by acknowledging in a straightforward way that the client's fearfulness is understandable and human because it "fits" the circumstances; and the counselor can well understand how frightening the prospect of going blind can be.

The counselor needs to listen perceptively so as to hear the "music" too. The music here is the underlying terror at being utterly helpless. Perhaps even medical or surgical interventions cannot forestall blindness—perhaps nothing can be done about that. But the counselor *can* deal with the issue of what can be done about being helpless, about feeling totally dependent, feeling useless. This fear can be dealt with in an affirmative way because many blind persons simply are not helpless, totally dependent, or useless. The counselor's qualities of warmth, empathy, and genuineness will very clearly have a direct effect in establishing that kind of trusting relationship by which this client can be helped to master her panic and move on to more positive, rational, and constructive behavior.

Plans and Problems in Counselor Training

Theoretically, at least, all the aforementioned characteristics can be developed through systematic, intensive training procedures. Aspiring peer counselors who do not appear to have good listening skills may yet, all else being equal, acquire these skills as part of their behavioral repertoire. On the other hand, practical considerations of limitations of time and energies available to the trainer may make the development of empathy, warmth, and genuineness in the trainee not at all feasible. This judgment will depend upon whether or not the social and interpersonal history of the trainee, his or her personality dynamics, attitudes, or other circumstances present overwhelming obstacles to success (or even acceptable progress) in the training process. Clearly it would be a prudent strategy to make the selection of peer counselors contingent upon satisfactory performance during the training sequence and through a predetermined probationary period. And this must be made explicit to each candidate for peer counseling training.

Experience as well as necessity requires that training peer counselors be as task-oriented as possible. This is based on the premise that good practice invariably is based upon good (valid) theory. I am simply emphasizing that for practical reasons the training of peer counselors need not and should not become mired in theoretical formulations burdened with philosophical abstractions and endless "picky" critiques of equivocal research or irrelevant case studies. First of all, such presentations will soon pall and bore the trainee who has an enthusiastic interest in how to do it. Second, while training so presented may appear to be the more sophisticated technique, the net effect may well turn out to be counterproductive. That is, such training may raise needless fears and anxieties about the complexities of that which the trainee seeks to do. Just such apprehensions have been known to frighten off very capable and potentially very effective peer counselors.

I do not mean to suggest that very real difficulties inherent in the counseling process should be denied or ignored in the training process. Difficulties, conflicts, and tensions which will most probably be encountered must be anticipated, confronted, and discussed in training sessions. Otherwise a partially prepared peer counselor is quite likely to be caught off guard and taken by surprise when a commonly encountered difficult circumstance does arise. Ill-prepared peer counselors are most vulnerable to feelings of inadequacy and uncertainty. If overwhelmed by such unpleasant feelings, they are the ones who are most likely to be irretrievably discouraged and who may well discontinue.

The dilemma for trainers of peer counselors, then, is to anticipate likely problems in such a way that the trainee will not later be inordinately surprised and discouraged. At the same time the trainer must avoid confronting the trainee with virtually every difficult contingency that can possibly be forecast. Escaping the horns of this dilemma in time-limited, intensive training depends in part on the trainer's experience but also on becoming familiar with, and sensitive to, the experiences, personality makeup, and strengths and weaknesses of individual trainees.

Outline of the Training Format

There is no one sure-fire, guaranteed formula for success in terms of training format. Training can be organized in a variety of ways, each of which, geared to specific intended outcomes, can be equally appropriate and effective. My own experience has been that all of the following stages, in this approximate order of steps, are important, interrelated components in training peers:

1. Discussion of goals in counseling
2. Presentation of facts about aging and the elderly
3. Learning to listen for and recognize feelings (the "music")
4. Learning to listen to and understand content (the "lyrics")
5. Developing a repertoire of appropriate responses to the client

6. Experiential (applied) training exercises
7. Follow-up and supervision.

Discussion of Goals

Given the frequently observed lack of specificity and clarity with respect to setting goals in counseling even among some experienced counselors, intiating early discussions with peer counselor trainees on goals is clearly a sensible training strategy. Whose goals, whose values, whose life-style, where responsibilities for decision-making rest—all these are matters of paramount importance and require considerable attention right at the beginning. This is particularly true of trainees who may approach the task with a built-in bias that counseling revolves around persuading the counselee to "do the right thing" or to "make the right decision." If trainees can themselves be convinced that counseling does not consist merely in advice-giving then virtually half the job is accomplished.

Presentation of Facts

One simply cannot assume that because candidates are themselves older persons they are without bias or stereotypic thinking about the aging process. We know that more than a few elderly do subscribe to at least some such myths, and the training process should demythologize aging for them. Peers need to begin their counseling armed with straight facts and reasonably unbiased attitudes about such pertinent issues as sexual activity, capability, and need in late life; intelligence, as well as learning capacity and performance of the aged; the extent to which behavior is affected by sensory changes and environmental factors; and the adaptive capabilities of older persons. Therefore, a succinct overview of facts about psychological, social, and physical aspects of the aging process has a most important and necessary place at this step in training. Candid discussion of such facts about aging will go a long way toward unmasking stereotypic views and attitudes, which can be dealt with.

Learning to Listen for and Recognize Feelings

Listening to the "message" of the client in counseling might be compared to listening to a song. The affect (feeling, tone) is analogous to listening to the music. The most effective peer counselor is one who has learned to recognize and understand the gamut of feelings which clients experience and bring with them into the counseling session. If it is indeed true that humans are most inclined to act on the basis of their feelings rather than on the basis of rationality, especially in relationships, then learning to listen for the music may be the most critical skill of all.

But feelings (the music) more often than not are expressed nonverbally: inflection and tones of voice, facial expression, body movements, and the like. Feelings are expressed also through other kinds of behaviors: dependability in keeping appointments, punctuality or tardiness, personal neatness or sloppiness, what one wears, where the client chooses to sit or stand in the office, etc. All these provide significant messages—clues, at least—as to what the client is feeling, perhaps thinking. The trainee must learn to become cognizant of, and in due course familiar with, such modes of communicating the music.

Learning to Listen to and Understand Content

Obviously the lyrics, too, make the song. And so the peer counselor candidate needs to attend to spoken words (the lyrics, to complete the analogy). Words spoken by the client are the symbols which tell the counselor, sooner or later, what the client's values and goals truly are. Words may not necessarily identify the crux of the problem or the underlying source of distress and pain and hurt. But the peer counselor must learn to recognize and understand words as signposts which point directions for relevant counseling.

Lyrics and music, that is, words and feelings: quite evidently two sides of the same communication coin. As a matter of strategy I would prefer to focus attention *first* on the affect dimension and subsequently on content. The reason is simple. Most persons are accustomed to attend automatically to words and may inadvertently miss the feelings. No doubt this is true of most trainees. Drawing attention first in the training sequence to feelings tends to create a set in the minds of trainees to weigh feelings at least equally on balance when assessing feeling/content aspects of the client's presentations.

It bears repeating that training needs to be practical, that is to say, easily translatable into practice. Well-devised and prepared exercises make this a reality. This leads, then, to the fifth step in training, which is:

Developing a Repertoire of Appropriate Response

Exercises in listening to and understanding the presentations of the client are needed at this stage. Candidates will benefit hugely from repeated opportunities to listen to actual presentations of clients. Prepared scripts (from case studies) are useful for this purpose and probably serve best as a beginning. Tapes of voices are even better because they are real-life events insofar as voice intonation, inflection, and expression are heard. Videotapes (with sound) are to be preferred if possible because they most nearly replicate real-life situations. A distinct advantage of videotapes is that the course of the presentation can be controlled (interrupted, replayed) for discussion, an option not available when observing live counseling sessions. The purpose of these exercises is to give the trainee practice in listening to the client and trying to identify and understand the client's communications.

Experiential (Applied) Training Exercises

One major training step yet needs to be considered: That is to train the aspiring peer counselor to develop a repertoire of appropriate verbal and nonverbal therapeutic responses.

How quickly and comfortably trainees acquire this necessary repertoire depends upon the qualities of empathy, warmth, and genuineness which they bring into training. We can predict that the level of competence already developed in recognizing and identifying a client's lyrics and music should facilitate each trainee's own self-expression and self-disclosure.

Most training programs appear calculated to help the learner examine his or her own verbal responses to the client. That is a necessary and useful function of training. Equally important and perhaps more difficult, however, is the task of helping the novice counselor become aware of and examine his nonverbal responses as well. The peer counselor must learn to assess his or her entire response repertoire in counseling (voice tone, inflection, facial expression, body posture, etc.) in terms of utility and appropriateness.

This task has at least two aspects. One is to train the candidate to see himself or herself as a stimulus to which the client responds in counseling. The counselor is no more a "blank page" than is the counselee. The counseling session is a here-and-now situation, and what takes place is contingent upon the kind and quality of interaction between the actors in that mini-drama. Therefore, training must make it clear that the peer-counselor-as-stimulus becomes a most significant variable in determining how the process evolves and whether or not a truly working, therapeutic relationship is developed.

The second aspect of this task is to assist the trainee to present a consistently warm, accepting (not identical to "agreeing"), straightforward empathic *persona* to the client. At the same time the trainee needs to learn how to avoid violating the client's personal sense of rationality and sensitivity. In other words, the trainee will be learning to respond to the client in ways that help the client maintain his sense of existential validation.

Case Examples

Mrs. Mandler. Mrs. Mandler, a 68-year-old widow with a pitiful, forlorn look about her, sits down with her counselor. She says to the counselor, "I am so terribly lonely since my husband died six years ago," and with that she begins to weep. It is evident that Mrs. Mandler is in great pain and distress. At all costs the counselor, an active, involved, usually cheerful person herself, must avoid the temptation to respond to Mrs. Mandler in a cheery voice with the observation, "Mrs. Mandler, there is simply no need for you to continue to be lonely and isolated and depressed. There are so many senior citizens' activities and clubs available to you out there."

By so responding the counselor in effect conveys to Mrs. Mandler the impression that she is somehow strange, perhaps a little incompetent in her feelings and in managing her life, that she is somehow unusual in feeling lonely and isolated. It may well be that Mrs. Mandler need not be burdened by the sense of loneliness as she is, but it is not therapeutic to add to her burden of hurt the notion that she is strange because she has those feelings. Much better would be a response that begins with, "I understand how you can feel that way, and I can tell how much you are hurting. I know how hard this can be. But let's get into this and see what we can do together."

Mrs. Critchberg. Mrs. Critchberg, age 72 years, tells her counselor a fascinating story of how she has worked for years as a legal secretary. She has also for many years lived singly, that is, until a young man, a law student from a school upstate, came into the office to work as a "paralegal" for one year. She tells of an affair between the two which she describes as one of the most intense turn-on experiences of her life. At the end of the year the law student left town to return to school. "Since that time," Mrs. Critchberg insists, "I have become a sex maniac. That's all I ever think of. And it is driving me out of my mind."

Again, the peer counselor must at all costs avoid reinforcing Mrs. Critchberg's own negative judgment of herself. She must avoid telling her client (even in a kindly fashion) "act your age." The counselor must make it explicit that she can understand her client's preoccupation with erotic feelings, that they are not absurd in a 72-year-old, and now that these long dormant sexual urges have been reawakened by the affair, her major problem seems to be finding an available, willing partner.

Commentary. Obviously the point here is that the trainer should explore the whole range of response options available to peer counselor trainees: restating client verbalizations (so they can hear how it sounds when said by the counselor), mirroring the feelings as perceived by the counselor ("You sound very angry about this"), interpreting the client's responses ("It seems to me that underneath it all you are very disappointed in your daughter"), confronting the client ("You seem to avoid facing up to what you said must be done"), summarizing the client's troubles or the client's options, exploring the consequences which can be expected in choosing a given option, and probing for more information ("Tell me more about what you said and how you were feeling when you said it").

As was the case with earlier steps in training, applicable exercises are very useful and productive in assisting the trainee to see himself or herself as a stimulus. Well-written scripts, for example, provide an excellent tool for eliciting responses from counselor trainees which can in turn be candidly and fairly critiqued through extensive discussion. The reading and discussion of carefully selected case studies provide the same opportunities. Another excellent training device is the use of role-playing, first by trainees with the experienced trainer, who provides a role model, then by trainees with each other.

Opportunities for gaining increased competence in appropriate and relevant self-disclosure is also an important part of this training step. The trainee certainly needs to be cautioned against using the counseling process for his or her own personal ends. That is, the peer counselor enjoys no license to burden the client with the counselor's own personal problems, difficulties, or fears. Nevertheless, there are times in the counseling process when it is relevant for the counselor to share personal feelings and/or experiences. When that kind of self-disclosure is done appropriately, it has a powerfully positive impact upon the counselee. Through sensitivity training, the peer counselor can learn to self-disclose comfortably and therapeutically.

A videotape of the role-playing, as already suggested, while not essential, has proved to be a most effective, powerful training tool. Trainees see their own behavioral responses in a way that is otherwise rarely if ever available to them. Here again, videotapes can be stopped and a particular segment reviewed and replayed without changing the sequence of events that ordinarily occur without interruption.

Follow-Up and Supervision

One last important element in training should be noted. Peer counselors of the elderly in most cases need a great deal of feedback, not only during the training, but also during post-training activity. Experience has shown that most peer counselors feel tenuous about their counseling work once they begin to do it with real clients, often because of fear of making some serious mistake. It is therefore a matter of critical importance that some experienced supervision be available during the post-training period. This should continue until the peer counselor has gained the confidence that comes from his prior experience. The feedback from a supervisor will of necessity be informational and corrective in some instances. In other instances feedback will consist of reassurance that the peer counselor is doing effective counseling. Some of this will come from the clients themselves, of course. But the counselors who stick with it are the ones sustained by the knowledge that the trainer or supervisor is "by their side" through those early days of doing peer counseling on their own.

Recommended Readings

Alpaugh, P. and Haney, M. *Counseling the older adult—a training manual.* Los Angeles: Andrus Center, University of Southern California, 1978.

Carp, F. The realities of interdisciplinary approaches: can the disciplines work together to help the aged? In A. N. Schwartz and I. Mensh (Eds.), *Professional obligations and approaches to the aged.* Springfield, Ill.: Charles C Thomas, 1974.

Kastenbaum, R. The reluctant therapist. In R. Kastenbaum, (Ed.), *New thoughts on old age.* New York: Springer, 1964.

Schwartz, A. N. and Peterson, J. A. *Introduction to gerontology.* New York: Holt, Rinehart and Winston, 1979.

Truax, C. and Carkhuff, R. *Toward effective counseling and psychotherapy: training and practice.* Chicago, Ill: Aldine, 1967.

Part III

Pathways to Behavior and Personality Change

10

The Humanistic Approach: The Ventura County Creative Aging Workshops

Richard A. Reinhart and S. Stansfeld Sargent

Beginnings of Humanistic Psychology

In 1954 a book called *Motivation and Personality* was published by a psychologist, Abraham H. Maslow. It contained a description and discussion of *self-actualizing people,* which occasioned a great deal of interest and excitement (Maslow, 1954). A few years later self-actualization became the central theme of a new trend or movement known as "humanistic psychology."

Humanistic psychologists thought of themselves as a "third force," to distinguish their program from psychoanalysis on the one hand and behaviorism on the other. They were centrally concerned with capacities and potentialities which they felt had been neglected, such as creativity, love, higher values, growth, spontaneity, humor, and self-actualization in general. Among those who joined Maslow in the new group were Carl Rogers, famous for his nondirective therapy; Rollo May, a foremost "existential" psychologist; Charlotte Bühler, internationally known developmental psychologist; and Sidney Jourard, becoming renowned for his emphasis on self-disclosure. Others prominent in psychology and related fields became active during the 1960s, writing for the publications and speaking at meetings sponsored by the new Association for Humanistic Psychology.

Maslow had earlier criticized his fellow psychologists for having far too limited a view of what the human being can attain. He felt that psychologists (and of course psychiatrists) had concentrated on the negative side—on human shortcomings, illnesses, and sins—and paid little attention to people's potentialities, virtues, and achievable aspirations.

Maslow's own emphasis contrasted sharply with this discouraging viewpoint. He stressed the strengths, the healthy component found in each person. He studied many famous persons (e.g., Lincoln, Jefferson, Einstein, Beethoven, Thoreau, Whitman, Schweitzer, Eleanor Roosevelt) and a number of his friends and acquaintances who were, as he put it, people who seemed to be "fulfilling themselves and to be doing the best that they are capable of doing." He analyzed the characteristics of this group of "self-actualizing people" and found several outstanding features which he described. One was a realistic emphasis; they accept themselves and their fellows and all of nature. They see human nature as it is and are not disgusted with the biological side of life, including the inevitable process of growing old. They are spontaneous and simple. Anything but egocentric, they are likely to become interested in projects which involve helping others. They love and identify with a small number of close friends, but do not seem to have time for a large circle of friends and acquaintances. They show continuing enjoyment of love, beauty, sex; they appreciate a sunset, flowers, babies, their own marriage. For them the business of daily living can be exciting. In fact, they report frequent ecstatic experiences or peaks of feeling, with wonder and awe, which have transformed and strengthened their daily lives. These could occur in milder forms many times a day. (See Maslow, 1968, Chapters 6 and 7.) And a sense of humor was definitely present in self-actualizing people, but it was of a philosophical and unhostile character, like the humor of Abe Lincoln. They might even make fun of themselves!

Probably the most universal characteristic of all the persons Maslow studied was creativeness, originality, or inventiveness in one or another area. It is not restricted to the arts or the intellect; there can be creative shoemakers, carpenters, or cooks. He thought of this quality as akin to the creativeness of unspoiled children—a potential given to all humans at birth, which is lost as they become "enculturated." Self-actualizing people need privacy and detachment.

They like solitude and are not dependent upon continual stimulation; they may be called "self-contained"—which others might interpret as coldness or snobbishness. They are not especially rebellious or unconventional, but operate according to the laws of their own character rather than the rules of society. This is likely to occasion some strain, but Maslow felt that a person can be healthy in our culture through a combination of inner autonomy and outer acceptance.

Maslow also noted other characteristics in his sample; e.g., more democratic values, a humility and readiness to learn from anybody, and a strong ethical sense. Self-actualizing people are by no means perfect; they can be vain, irritating, or uncritical, and they are not free from guilt, anxiety, and conflict. However, they are mature and are both more individual and more completely socialized. In a word, they have resolved the common conflicts between heart and head, acceptance and rebellion, introversion and extroversion.

Self-actualizing people, Maslow insisted, are the foundation for a positive science of psychology; they suggest the heights which people can attain. Neurosis is basically the failure of personal growth. The job of a psychologist or counselor is to help clients unfold and develop, and to get to know and accept themselves.

Persons who wish to actualize themselves might or might not be the kind who are considered "neurotic" or "mentally ill." Their peers might even think of them as "well-adjusted" or "superior." Their common characteristic is simply a desire to improve and fulfill themselves, to grow, to realize their own potential. They can be rich or poor, well or poorly educated, foreign or native-born, male or female, and young, middle-aged, or old.

Let's Not Overlook Individual Differences!

We must remember that the individual differences found among older people are, if anything, greater than those found in any other age group. As one of the pioneers in gerontology, Ollie Randall, commented in regard to the aging and the aged:

> We are perhaps the most individualistic people alive today. We are no longer conformists, as we were apt to be when we were younger, unless we are compelled to be by circumstances beyond our control. We are as different from one another as it is possible to be, even when we belong to the same family or the same culture [Randall, 1977].

She added that the differences are accentuated further by variations in retirement, illness, the higher death rates of men than of women, the inroads of inflation, and many other factors.

This is an important dash of realism, because it is only too easy to speak about "old people," "the aging," "the elderly," etc., as if they were all alike. Such sloppy thinking can easily result in confused action.

Psychologically speaking, there are at least three major groups among our senior citizens. At one extreme are the well-adjusted, highly motivated, more or less self-actualizing people, who are seldom in need of help. At the other extreme we find the isolated, often inaccessible persons who are heard from only when they are in dire straits. In between is a larger segment of the older population who are independent, sociable, fairly well-adjusted and active—in a word, the "normal" or "average" people.

Actually some of this middle group, though unfamiliar with the principles of humanistic psychology, are found to be applying tenets of self-actualization in their daily lives. Many have learned to accept themselves as older people, to live a simpler life, and to become closer to nature. Some retirees are more detached and private than they used to be, and are pleased about it rather than feeling lonely or alienated. Many have become more independent of cultural pressures and do not feel as much need to conform as they formerly did. In their later years quite a few people come to feel closer to friends and relatives and seek to renew old ties that have become weak.

But we must be careful not to distort a very complex picture. In contrast to the above, older people frequently show a loss of spontaneity and creativity. Many become dependent and self-centered, more complaining, increasingly lacking in sense of humor whether due to illness or other causes. Some simply withdraw into TV, drugs, or alcohol.

Humanistic psychologists are challenged by this situation. They believe that many older people can be helped to retain the self-actualizing characteristics they have developed, or to regain at least some of the ones they have lost. And a few of them may even be inspired to acquire positive ways of living for the first time. Can this really be done?

Most of us who work with seniors can think of cases which illustrate self-actualization. An elderly widow of a professional man had become slightly confused and disorientated, so she had difficulty in riding buses and in getting around on the local college campus where she wanted to attend classes. She had a good mind and some education and was very frustrated unless she was involved in something intellectual. It was possible to help her find interesting courses given by the Santa Monica Emeritus College at locations within easy walking distance, so she could attend one class a day. This allayed her major frustrations and gave her intellectual stimulation and a sense of accomplishment.

Mrs. Riston, in her 70s, was depressed and anxious, with many somatic complaints. Since she had formerly held a job and been active in social organizations, the therapist looked for a way to restore her self-esteem. A Retired Senior Volunteer Program had just been established in the community, so she was referred to its director. There had been a delay in obtaining a secretary for the program so Mrs. Riston, as the first volunteer, served temporarily as the secretary, which she was well able to do because of her background in business. She played an important part in getting the new program off the ground and was very proud of being the first secretary and the "Number One Volunteer." Mrs. Riston later told a news reporter that the RSVP had changed her whole life and given her something to live for.

Several organizations now exist which have programs applying the principles and techniques of humanistic psychology for the benefit of persons over age 60. Probably the best known of these is SAGE (an acronym for Senior Actualization and Growth Explorations), founded in 1974 in Berkeley, California. It has been described as "a humanistically focused self-development program for men and women over 60 years of age" which has been "exploring the many ways in which the later years of life can be a time for health, vitality, expanded awareness, and the realization of self that comes from having lived a long and full life" (Dychtwald, 1978). SAGE uses many physical and mental training and therapeutic techniques similar to those developed at the Esalen Institute, the original humanistic psychology growth center. These include massage, yoga, sensory awareness, relaxation, meditation, breathing exercises, and biofeedback, along with group and individual counseling.

SAGE methods have been successful in increasing the health, emotional stability, and self-esteem of its elderly participants, according to the testimony of many of them. For example, one 73-year-old member who describes herself as "and old post-cancer case with high blood pressure" says:

> At SAGE I have been learning how to be alive and vital again. For example, I was recently at a party and ate some of the wrong things.

> When I went home, I suffered from a tachycardia [rapid heartbeat] attack. I immediately put myself into a state of deep relaxation and practiced yogic breathing and the attack quickly passed. . . . In addition to becoming more aware of myself in a physical way, I have also been learning quite a bit about my mind and my feelings. In my SAGE group I had a chance to work through some of my long-repressed grief about losing six people including my brother within a short period of time. One day I was doing my deep breathing exercises when emotions started coming up and I began to cry. . . . I wept bitterly for two hours, and I wept away a score of sorrows. And, finally, I started to laugh, thinking of all the people who have loved me all my life and still love me. . . . Thanks to SAGE, I'll never be the same. No one ever had a chance at age 73 to live a new life as I have [Dychtwald, 1978, p. 70].

The SAGE group has extended its therapeutic program into homes for the aged, nursing and rest homes, and convalescent hospitals in the Bay Area of California. Various kinds of training are offered for workers with the aging. SAGE has inspired the founding of similar types of programs in Hawaii, Florida, Denver, Los Angeles, Chicago, and other localities. Out of these activities has come a new organization, the Association for Humanistic Gerontology, designed to advance the ideas and methods of a humanistic approach to a study of the life and problems of older people.

Let us turn now to a county-wide program for the aging, organized along the lines of the positive approach of humanistic psychology.

Creative Aging Workshops in the Community

The setting up of Creative Aging Workshops in different communities of Ventura County (California) grew out of a concern on the part of several members of the Mental Health Department. The chief psychologist noted that, like the staffs of community mental health programs throughout the nation, the Ventura group had problems in trying to make their services known to and used by persons in their senior years. This national concern has been well documented and was the basis for the 1977 revisions of the Community Mental Health Centers Act which now mandates programs for seniors if communities are to receive federal funding.

In Ventura County, he said, our mental health staff faced the discouraging discovery that in the fiscal year 1976–77, only 2 percent or 243 persons in the active caseloads in all three of the county catchment areas consisted of persons over 65. This was true despite the fact that seniors constitute 10 percent of the county's population of 460,000 and that national estimates suggest that at any one time, at least 6 percent of seniors need mental health services (Kobrynski, 1975). Applied to the county figures, that would mean a disturbed senior population of almost 2,700. Our care provided to 243 persons meant that we were meeting only 9 percent of the estimated need.

Furthermore, of the 9,400 hours per year our staff devoted to community activities for consultation, information, education, and organization, only 6 percent or 520 hours were given to agencies and community groups concerned with the needs of seniors.

Why the wide discrepancy between the very considerable needs of seniors and the meager services supplied them? A major cause is undoubtedly the well-known resistance of older people to psychiatric and mental health treatment, which is discussed in other parts of this book. At the same time, many mental health workers feel uncomfortable with the idea of having seniors as clients. In some cases it is because workers feel inexperienced with elders. In other instances workers are concerned about difficulties they have heard about: older people are rigid and detest change; they have trouble gaining and using insight; they remain fixated on their symptoms, etc. (Butler, 1970).

It was clear that a major effort needed to be made to distribute our service capabilities so they included seniors more often. But how was this to be done? How could we address ourselves to the problems of resistance on the part of seniors to avail themselves of mental health help? And how could we promote more interest on the part of our staff to work with seniors?

Two other related questions occurred to us: Could we also function in a more preventive way—i.e., attracting older people not now distressed but eager to head off trouble in the future? And, in line with principles of humanistic psychology, could we not also serve perfectly "normal" seniors interested in learning more about themselves, in improving themselves—in a word, in self-actualization?

The first order of business seemed to be to learn who among our staff was interested in working with a senior population. A memo announcing the formation of a Creative Aging Committee went to each of the 180 professional staff of the Ventura County Mental Health Services. To that first organization meeting came about fifteen professionals: one psychiatrist, two psychologists, three social workers, three mental health nurses, three psychiatric technicians, and three rehabilitation therapists. These fifteen, representing about

9 percent of the full staff from each of the three regional catchment areas, constituted the core group of planners and "doers."

Next, we invited representatives of the agencies and organizations that relate to senior citizens, in order to get outside assessments of how mental health staff skills might best be employed in the community.

Out of these meetings grew the idea of a series of public workshops for seniors, each concerned with common emotional problems and human needs specific to the later years. To avoid the label of mental disorder and to widen the range of concerns to be dealt with, we decided to call the free public meetings Workshops on Creative Aging and to invite other organizations working with seniors to cosponsor the events and bring their unique perspectives to bear on the problem.

A task force to organize and plan the workshops was developed, consisting of Ventura County Mental Health Services professionals and representatives from eight other local organizations such as the Retired Senior Volunteer Program, Senior Survival Services of the county's Public Social Services Agency, the Hot Meals and Meals-on-Wheels program, the Adult Education Department of Ventura Unified School District, the Emeritus Program at Ventura College, and the Recreation Departments run by cities. In addition, an interested physician from the community expressed willingness to come and talk about nutrition concerns in later life.

Now the major question was, Where in the county should we have our first workshop?

County Planning Department census data provided the answer: Oak View, a small community of about 8,000 in the northwestern part of the county some fifteen miles from Ventura, had the largest concentration of persons over 60 years of age in the county.

Then we hit a new snag: Oak View had no public facilities capable of holding the 75 persons we had hoped might come to this first in the series on creative aging. Nor was there much hope of finding a building which provided relatively self-enclosed rooms for the seven or eight different subjects that were to be discussed.

A large church in Oak View heard of our dilemma and came forth to offer its facilities for the conference. It had both the small Sunday school rooms for the individual sessions we needed, plus the church itself for the plenary sessions.

One reason for the church's special interest, explained an officer of the congregation, was that the church membership included many seniors who might well benefit from the workshop. Would we also need their kitchen and dining hall facilities? they wanted to know.

That question sparked the idea of combining the workshop with a nutritious meal and extending the workshop to both morning and afternoon.

The task force pondered the problem of the relative isolation of Oak View as a site for this first conference.

The Recreation Department offered its buses, the other agencies their vehicles, and we soon had an operational motor pool to offer rides to seniors when needed.

The task force arranged for publicity around the entire county: news releases, radio interviews, posters printed and distributed to mobile park homes and senior housing areas, church bulletins, supermarket bulletin boards, recreation centers, anywhere and everywhere seniors might see it (see Fig. 1 and Fig. 2).

We asked people to register in advance, fearing we might have to cancel the whole idea if only a few seniors showed interest. Would they be frightened by the stereotype and the bugaboo of "mental health"? We offered a variety of topics, including physical fitness, nutrition and health, senior survival, and "love or loneliness." But would they appear and discuss such emotionally charged topics as "emotional ups and downs in the senior years," "human sexuality," "the woman alone," "alternatives to depression," and "death and dying"?

The answer was an overwhelming "YES!" To our amazement, seniors walked, drove, hobbled, and wheelchaired to the first Creative Aging Workshop in October 1977—150 of them—seriously stretching the church's capacity (and our credulity).

The program was planned so that each workshop was given in the morning and repeated in the afternoon. Thus, each participant could attend two sessions. They were asked to indicate four choices in order of preference and the choices were followed as closely as possible in planning the sessions.

Most came for the day, although a few stayed just for the morning, had their lunch, and left. During lunch, some of the workshop staff began plunking at a church piano. One or two added their voices when they recognized a song, and soon the seniors in the dining hall transformed the session into an old-fashioned community sing.

As pleasant as the social experience was (and individual workshop leaders made a special effort to spend time acquainting each person in the group with their neighbors on either side), it was the readiness with which many seniors brought out their problems of an intimate nature and spoke out their feelings despite the presence of others that surprised and moved the workshop staff.

The authors of this article co-led the workshop entitled "The

Figure 1. Creative Aging Registration Form.

CREATIVE AGING WORKSHOPS

Come and be with friends for a day of sharing and learning to live more effectively!

FREE

FOR: SENIORS

DATE: OCT. 19, 1977

FREE

TIME: 9 AM – 3:30 PM

PLACE: 195 MAHONEY AVE
OAK VIEW, CALIF.

LUNCH: 12 - 1:30 FURNISHED BY HOT MEALS

SPONSORS

COMMISSION ON HUMAN CONCERNS
COUNCIL ON AGING, VENTURA COUNTY/OJAI
FIRST BAPTIST CHURCH, OAK VIEW
HEALTH CARE AGENCY
ALCOHOL SERVICES
MENTAL HEALTH SERVICES
INTERESTED CITIZENS AND VOLUNTEERS
PARKS & RECREATION DEPTS.,
THOUSAND OAKS & VENTURA
SENIOR NUTRITION PROGRAM
SENIOR SURVIVAL SERVICES
STATE DEPARTMENT OF HEALTH
TRI-COUNTIES AREA AGENCY ON AGING
VENTURA UNIFIED SCHOOL DISTRICT

REGISTRATION FORM

NAME ______________________________

ADDRESS ______________________________

PHONE ____________________

CREATIVE AGING
OCTOBER 19, 1977
9 A.M.-3:30 P.M.
195 MAHONEY AVENUE
OAK VIEW, CA.

INDICATE BELOW YOUR CHOICES FOR THE WORKSHOPS. PLEASE USE THE NUMBERS PRECEDING EACH WORKSHOP DESCRIPTION.

FIRST ________ THIRD ________

SECOND ________ FOURTH ________

MAIL TO:
JUNE ARBER
COMMUNITY SERVICES/MH
300 HILLMONT AVENUE
VENTURA, CA 93003

Figure 2. Creative Aging Agenda.

** CREATIVE AGING WORKSHOP **

9:00-9:30 a.m.	Registration and Coffee Jane Funeg & Jane Coffman
9:30-10:00 a.m.	Welcome Address June Arber
10 a.m.-12 noon	WORKSHOPS
12 noon-1:30 p.m.	Lunch Break
1:30 p.m.-3:30 p.m.	WORKSHOPS

****

Please select four choices from the workshops below and list them in order of preference in the space provided on the registration form on back. We will let you know at the workshop which two sessions you may attend. Hopefully these will be your first choices.

1. EMOTIONAL UPS AND DOWNS IN THE SENIOR YEARS
This workshops asks you to look at ideas and expectations of how people in their 60's, 70's and 80's are "supposed" to feel. Your experiences with this and how it contrasts with how you actually feel will be part of the workshop. Richard Reinhart & Stan Sargent

2. THE WOMAN ALONE
There will be discussion of problems facing the unmarried older woman in today's society. A sharing experience! Barbara Young & Colleen House

3. ALTERNATIVES TO DEPRESSION
This group will teach how to be more assertive as a way to prevent depression. Exercises will be aimed at enhancing self-awareness, self-esteem and communication skills. Genie Wheeler and Barbara Childers

4. SENIOR SUNSHINE
This workshop deals with different approaches to senior physical fitness in everyday living, with live demonstrations, as well as slides and tapes from the T.V. show, "Senior Sunshine Fitness Factory." Barbara Weed & Associates

5. LOVE OR LONELINESS
This workshop will help us to understand the nature of loneliness and how love can replace it. Practical techniques will be taught and relaxation exercises will be demonstrated as an aid in self-awareness. Doyle Shields, Erma Holloway, Barbara Loubek

6. DEATH AND DYING
This workshop is designed to help participants examine their own values and beliefs about death, dying and grieving, as well as to provide current information. Mary Lee Hogeback and Rita Reuben

7. HUMAN SEXUALITY
This workshop is dedicated to people who wish both to better understand their own sexual needs and behavior, and to be more accepting of their neighbor whose sexual attitudes and behavior might be different from their own. Gina Manchester & Rene Beauchesne

8. SENIOR SURVIVAL AND RESOURCES
A workshop about resources in the community for seniors who need it. Information and referral services to these helping agencies will be discussed. Ginny Gray & Tony Lamb

9. NUTRITION AND HEALTH
This workshop will provide valuable information on nutrition and related topics, such as maintaining an adequate nutritional balance, evaluating your diet, rating fast food service in regard to nutrition and special food bargains in the Ventura area. Dexter Weed

Emotional Ups and Downs of Later Life." In it, seniors began to share with evident emotion their own life crises in recent years. Some widows spoke of the intense feelings of loneliness after their husbands died. There was common agreement in the form of head-nodding and murmured assent when one told of her determination to avoid "burdening" others with her loneliness. Others expressed surprise in learning about resources available to them as residents of Ventura County. Still others shared what they had done to battle the common problems of isolation and transportation limitations. At the end of 90 minutes, most in the circle of 20 to 25 persons had taken at least one turn in bringing up a particular problem, making a suggestion to others, or commenting in one form or another.

Following individual sessions, persons attending all the workshops reconvened for the plenary session before lunch. Evaluation forms had been distributed at the conclusion of each workshop, and tables had been set up at exit points with signs requesting that completed evaluations be left in a designated box.

Of the 150 seniors attending, 93 completed questionnaires. There was nearly unanimous approval of the housekeeping aspects of the meeting—e.g., location, transportation, registration, luncheon. On the workshops proper, both the morning and afternoon sessions showed about the same results in terms of interest and stimulation, useful information, and degree of participation by the respondents as well as how they saw others participating. Overall, the workshops were highly rated, with about 75 percent of the evaluations being either in the "excellent" or the "good" category. Similarly, the individual workshops were all rated predominantly excellent or good.

Most of the comments and suggestions were also favorable, e.g.:

> Enjoyed them all. Would like to attend more.
>
> Workshops were excellent and gives one the opportunity of knowing others' problems and recognizing one's own.
>
> Come back again. Would like to take those I didn't take today.

Where there was criticism, it tended to be positive, e.g.:

> Workshops would be more helpful if more guidelines could be given by the instructor. Most persons are seeking answers that are perhaps disturbing to them.
>
> One hour sessions would be better.
>
> We only scratched the surface. Want more sessions like this.

Aside from the formal answers given in the questionnaire, workshop leaders without exception reported that many seniors had expressed their personal feelings of pleasure and gratitude for the workshop. Certificates of workshop completion were given to those who had registered and attended the event.

Newspaper coverage for the workshops was excellent, with favorable editorial comment in the local paper. The reporter gave some interesting sidelights on the sessions (McKean, 1977). One woman apparently got into the sexuality workshop by mistake and quickly left with the explanation "I'm not interested in sex at all." But twenty others disagreed. As one put it: "I was married for 25 years, divorced when I was 50, and I'm trying to make up my mind now about this whole aspect. . . ." Another said, "I'm a widow but I am also concerned with responsiveness and sexuality and I think I have a right to be." Most of the discussions were serious, but with a few lighter moments such as, in the session on death and dying, when a woman commented:

> My mother always told me to make sure my undergarments were clean so that if I was hauled into an emergency room to die, there wouldn't be dirty undies to mess it all up.

About six months after the Oak View meetings, a second conference was held in the eastern part of Ventura County, at Thousand Oaks. A similar series of workshops was offered and about 100 people participated. This one seemed to tap seniors with a higher socioeconomic standing, since many of them arrived in their own cars. A few had attended the first conference and had enjoyed it so much that when they read about the Thousand Oaks workshop, they decided to come and re-experience the pleasure and benefit the first had given them.

The next workshop was all in Spanish, with a new cadre of Spanish-speaking leaders. It was held in the agricultural community of Santa Paula, in the central part of the county. A somewhat different list of workshop topics was offered, including "death and dying," "dangerous drugs and alcohol," "how to use police help," and "what to do about depression." Almost 100 seniors appeared at the workshop, and there were many spontaneous expressions of pleasure and appreciation for the sessions, though no formal evaluation was attempted. Other workshops are planned for parts of the county not yet reached, using larger and more representative organizing committees.

They Support Each Other

Dr. Alice Dondero was a leader in the Ventura County Spanish-speaking Creative Aging Workshop. "One of the important things," she stated, "is that the seniors learned that they in fact do have some personal power to change things, and that they are not as isolated when they do things in groups. They support each other."

One person much helped by the workshop was José, a recently retired Mexican-American who had resisted being considered old, had refused to attend senior citizen activities, and had isolated himself from all but his family. Somehow his wife persuaded him to attend the workshop. There José watched a spontaneous *teatro* (skit) showing a depressed and lonely man being invited to come to a senior center. The man declines, giving excuses, crying, "No, no, no!" to all appeals. But he finally yields, and as the skit closes he is warming up to the laughter and pleasant society of the clubhouse.

The message got through to José. He now comes regularly to his neighborhood center for seniors, where he socializes, plays games, and even attends classes and group meetings. Now he can accept the label of *mayor* (senior or oldster) and enjoys being with others his own age. And to his own family he is a much nicer and happier *abuelo* (grandfather).

Overview of the Workshops

It is difficult to assess the overall effect of the Creative Aging Workshops at this time. Apparently, many participants have felt the sessions were generally enjoyable, broadening, and "self-actualizing," as suggested by the favorable comments made on the evaluation sheets. Some were even inspired to action; e.g., the senior who stated, "Useful to be in a group where some have had actual experience. If there are any services resulting from this workshop, I would be willing to visit people who are dying." On the other hand, some reactions suggest that participants were actually helped with personal problems, e.g., "Through the afternoon discussion I believe I have found an answer to my personal need."

One of the best indications of the success of these workshops and other projects involving members of the Mental Health Services' Creative Aging Committee is the fact that recent reexamination of the proportion of Ventura County clientele over age 60 has shown, in the past year, a doubling of the percentage of senior clients receiving direct treatment services in the form of individual and group or family therapy. And, in addition, more than 1,200 hours of indirect community services (consultation, education, information, and community organization) were offered to seniors and organizations that work with them around the county. This was more than double the number of hours given the previous year. Finally, the county training officer reports that more staff members have been signing up for training courses on working with seniors than has ever happened in the past.

Nor should we overlook the good feeling on the part of workshop leaders and their expressed willingness to prepare for and participate in future workshops. The chief psychologist summed it up this way: "We get better and better at the organization of these events, and our confidence has grown that, despite our fears, the subject of emotional problems and the resources for help that are available in the county for seniors is of intense interest to them."

Recommended Readings

Brammer, L. M. and Shostrom, E. L. *Therapeutic psychology: fundamentals of actualization counseling and psychotherapy* (2nd ed.). Englewood Cliffs, N.J.: Prentice-Hall, 1968.

Bugental, J. F. T. (Ed.). *Challenges of humanistic psychology.* New York: McGraw-Hill, 1967.

Buhler, C. and Allen, M. *Introduction to humanistic psychology.* Monterey, CA: Brooks/Cole, 1972.

Jourard, S. *Personal adjustment: an approach through the study of healthy personality* (2nd ed.) New York: Macmillan, 1963.

Maslow, A. H. *Motivation and personality.* New York: Harper and Row, 1954; Rev. ed., 1970.

Maslow, A. H. *Toward a psychology of being* (2nd ed.) Princeton, N.J.: Van Nostrand, 1968.

Sargent, S. S. The humanistic approach to personality, *in* Wolman, B. B. (Ed.). *Handbook of general psychology.* Englewood Cliffs, N.J.: Prentice-Hall, 1973.

11

Behavioral Approaches to Therapy with the Elderly

Jeffrey C. Rosenstein and Edwin W. Swenson

What is a chapter on behavioral approaches doing in a book on *nontraditional* approaches to counseling and psychotherapy? The notions upon which the behavioral model is based were articulated as long ago as the time of Rousseau. Behaviorism has held a prominent place in systematic psychology for over a half century and can be found in one guise or another in every storehouse of *tradition* the discipline has to offer. Behavior modification became a household term nearly a decade ago when B. F. Skinner's controversial *Beyond Freedom and Dignity* (1971) became a best-seller. Since then, the fuss seems to have abated, and the whole business has been well assimilated into the fabric of everyday life. By now, behavioral approaches certainly appear to have all the markings of tradition.

Yet, while behavioral approaches have carved out their own niches in history, in academic psychology, and in mainstream society, they have been rather slow to enter into clinical practice. Today they are widely accepted and applied by clinicians, but less so in working with the elderly population (Hoyer, Mishara, and Riebel, 1975). Moreover the modest number of published behavioral approaches to treatment of the elderly focuses primarily on the problems of severely disturbed, institutionalized individuals (Kahn and Zarit, 1974; Kahn, 1975, 1977). Most certainly, applications of the behavioral model in other settings, to other problems, and with other elderly people have yet to be tried, evaluated, and reported. Lindsley (1964) pointed out that, in spite of behavior modification programs for other populations, no such programs exist for older persons. He charged that society had not made use of scientific findings to construct appropriate supporting environments for the aged. Since Lindsley's challenge in 1964, the situation has remained essentially the same (Brink, 1979). Studies have been attempted on a somewhat limited scale to use a behavioral approach with older persons (Swenson, 1965; Cautela and Kastenbaum, 1967; Libb and Clements, 1969; Cautela, 1969; Davison, 1969; Lawton and Gottesman, 1974), but have not dealt with the complex prosocial and living skills necessary to counteract the problems of acquired dependence, withdrawal, and depression. "Behavior modification techniques constitute a natural, but almost unexplored, area of intervention on behalf of the elderly" (Lawton and Gottesman, 1974, p. 690). Hence, for now, the word *nontraditional* may be understating the nature and extent of the practice of behavioral treatment methods in clinical gerontopsychology.

A nontraditional approach is not necessarily good. In the realm of counseling and psychotherapy with the aged, however, the traditional approach has clearly failed to demonstrate the same effect it seems to have when working with younger persons. This failure can be traced to two general factors: (1) the model of service delivery demanded by the traditional approach and (2) the particular characteristics of the target population and its problems. If we do not pursue alternatives, such as the behavioral model, we are forced to work within the constraints of the traditional approach and achieve, at best, limited success.

The constraints imposed by the model of service delivery, which follows along the guidelines of the traditional medical model, are especially restrictive. First, there is an underlying presupposition that persons in need of treatment are, in some way, diseased or maladjusted. Generally, the problems requiring treatment must have reached crisis proportions before contact with the service provider is made. The nature of the contact with the service provider is highly formalized and institutionalized, requiring travel to an office, a hospital, or a mental health center. Once contact has been made, treatment is generally provided on a one-to-one basis by a highly trained professional. The cost of the treatment is generally high. The time-course of treatment may be quite lengthy.

The problems raised by these constraints are numerous. It is stigmatizing for an individual to receive treatment. There is little attention directed to preventive measures; hence, only highly visible and severely disabling problems receive treatment. The individual or his family must generally initiate the contact with a service provider and must be mobile enough to avail himself or herself of the services offered. There must be a sufficient number of trained professionals to meet the demand for service. The individual must have sufficient financial resources to pay for treatment and may often be required to invest a substantial amount of time in order to reap its benefits.

The constraints imposed by the target population are, perhaps, even more restrictive and interact with the problems stemming from the traditional model of service delivery. Elderly persons are, generally, especially sensitive to the stigma of treatment. Any service identified as psychotherapy or counseling is often avoided both because of its label, which carries a dim but ever-present allusion to exorcism of evil spirits, and for what it represents: that the individual is ill and incapable of independent functioning. The vast majority of the aged population lives independently, in small communities, where the stigma of mental health treatment is especially great, and where the only alternative to fully independent living is institutionalization.

Most elderly persons live on restricted incomes and cannot afford or are unwilling to pay for high-priced services in the private sector. If community services are available, they are often avoided because they are highly visible. Additionally, most community mental health centers do not provide services specifically tailored to the needs of the aged, even though they are mandated by the federal government to do so. Moreover, services that are provided in community mental health centers are generally administered by young persons (under 35 years of age), with whom the elderly feel little rapport. Of course, the individual seeking treatment must be able to travel to the place it is provided. For persons who do not drive or who live in a community without good public transportation, this is another obstacle to receiving treatment.

The presenting problems of the elderly population are, for the most part, no different from any other, but the frequency with which some are represented is clearly disproportionate. Then, there are some problems which are seemingly exclusively the problems of old age. Many of these difficulties seem to stem from problems in daily living. Such situations as coping with retirement, interacting with social service agencies, learning to deal with adult children and very aged parents, living on a restricted income, coping with sensorimotor and memory deficits, living with a progressively diminishing number of contemporaries, and adjusting to increasingly more complex technology are some of the difficulties that are fairly idiosyncratic to the aged population. Psychodynamic approaches, while often helpful, were not especially designed to assist with problems of this nature.

Characteristics of the Behavioral Approach

The behavioral approach offers a viable treatment alternative which does not require the traditional medical model of service delivery. Behavioral interventions have as their goal the restructuring of an individual's interactions with his environment and the people who live in it. Hence, they deal directly with specific situations and problems experienced by the person receiving treatment, rather than intrapsychic entities. The orientation of the behavioral approach is educational. Through systematic training, it assists persons in need in building and strengthening meaningful, adaptive, and appropriate personal and social behavior. With behavior change, people concomitantly develop greater self-esteem, socially desirable personality characteristics, greater sensitivity to and understanding of other persons, stronger and more rewarding interpersonal relationships, and a wider range of skills in coping with and mastering their environments.

Some characteristics of behavioral approaches which indicate that they may be particularly appropriate in meeting the needs of older persons are as follows:

1. The objectives utilized are specific and operational. There are no mysterious or magical entities postulated, and the entire therapeutic process may be readily explained to and be understood by the client.

2. The emphasis is on the use of positive, rather than aversive techniques. The treatment process is deliberately constructed to be rewarding to the client, thus maximizing the client's motivation to participate fully in and succeed at the tasks required.

3. Paraprofessionals as well as professionals can readily use the techniques. Hence, the number and variety of persons able to provide services to the target population is greatly increased.

4. The approaches are relatively brief and economical. The cost of treatment is therefore reduced both in terms of dollars and in the behavioral commitment required on the part of the client. Gains are generally seen more quickly; hence, consumer satisfaction is frequently high.

5. They can be understood and utilized by and with persons from a variety of socioeconomic and educational backgrounds. Because behavioral approaches focus on the *process* of learning, rather than on the language, extent, or content of learning per se, they tap an element of common human experience. The concepts and mechanics of behavioral approaches are simple, straightforward, and easily articulated.

6. They are effective in dealing with a wide variety of problems. The literature of behavior therapy is rapidly expanding, with literally thousands of successful applications of behavioral principles to specific problems reported. These applications range from teaching such basic skills as grooming, eating, and dressing to such complex skills as effective parenting, increasing marital satisfaction, and financial planning. They have been utilized with institutionalized retarded persons and college-educated professionals.

7. They can be used in the natural environment. It is not necessary or even desired to have treatment take place away from the client's real, everyday world. Problems can be dealt with where they exist, rather than in a doctor's office, a hospital, or a mental health center. Because treatment can be provided at home, in schools, in community centers, in churches, etc., it is less stigmatizing to receive services, for they do not necessarily have to be identified as psychotherapeutic.

Behavioral approaches are founded upon the notion that a person's behavior and feelings are heavily influenced (and sometimes completely determined) by experience. If an individual's experience of the world and of himself is altered, then his behavior or feelings may change. Experience is assimilated through learning, with three types of learning basic to the behavioral approach.

Types of Learning

Classical conditioning postulates that behavior and feelings are *elicited* by certain stimuli (i.e., objects, situations, persons, etc.) that we have come to associate with similar responses through repeated experience. For example, if on several occasions a person experiences acute physical distress (e.g., pain) while in the presence of another particular person (e.g., a dentist), a very strong association between the two will develop. Then, whenever the dentist is encountered, even if it is in a social situation having nothing to do with the drilling and filling of teeth, a person will feel distressed at the sight of the dentist and act to avoid him. Sometimes stimuli and responses may become strongly associated the very first time they are experienced together (Guthrie, 1952). But in general the strength of association grows with repeated similar experience.

In operant conditioning, behavior and feelings are postulated to be affected by their *consequences,* unlike classical conditioning, which states that behavior and feelings are controlled by *antecedent* stimuli. The operant learning paradigm assumes that, for numerous reasons, we respond in particular ways to objects, people, and situations. These responses *emitted* are termed *operants.* Following the emission of an operant, the individual may experience one of two types of stimuli (consequences): a *reinforcer* or a *punisher.* Or the person may experience nothing at all, a consequence termed *extinction.*

A reinforcer is, by definition, a consequence which strengthens (increases) the behavior which preceded it. Reinforcers are generally experienced as pleasurable events or rewarding objects (i.e., a compliment, a hug from a loved one, a good-tasting meal, a trip to a favorite place, etc.) These types of stimuli are positive reinforcers. Reinforcers may also be experienced as relief from unpleasant experience (i.e., cessation of pain or discomfort, leaving a noxious place, having a distressing object or person removed, etc.). These consequences are termed negative reinforcers. Both positive and negative reinforcers strengthen (increase) the behavior which precede them. Hence, the behavior will tend to be emitted more frequently, with greater intensity, with a shorter latency, or for a longer period of time.

A punisher is a consequence which suppresses the behavior which preceded it. Punishers are usually experienced as unpleasant events or objects (i.e., criticism, pain or physical distress, removal of a previously acquired reinforcer, etc.). When punishers are experienced as the consequence of certain behaviors, those behaviors tend to be emitted less readily, less frequently, with less intensity, with a greater latency, or for a shorter period of time. Note, however, that these behaviors *are still emitted.*

If a behavior is emitted repeatedly, with no discernible consequences whatsoever (i.e., it is completely ignored, results in no reinforcers, or results in no punishers, etc.), this is a condition termed *extinction.* Extinction *removes* the behavior which precedes it from the repertoire of behaviors emitted.

If a person receives repeated and enraptured attention (a reinforcer) for telling a particular story, that story will tend to be told more frequently and may become progressively embellished with each telling. If, on the other hand, at its conclusion, people consistently remark that it was uninteresting or boring (a punisher), it will tend to be repeated less frequently and may become progressively shorter with each telling. If people do not respond at all and go about their business as if the story had not been told (extinction), the story will tend not to be repeated again.

Complex or difficult behaviors are acquired by experiencing reinforcers for successive closer approximations of the desired behavior. This is a process called *shaping.* Therefore, when learning to play golf, it is at first reinforcing merely to hit the ball with the club and have it travel anywhere. Then, after having learned to connect with the ball repeatedly, one is reinforced only when it travels down the fairway toward the green. After learning to avoid playing in the rough, one is reinforced only by moving the ball from the tee to the hole in fewer and fewer strokes. Eventually, it becomes reinforcing to approach or to break par. This is an example of shaping. To expect a beginner to break par is absurd, as it is equally ridiculous to expect a seasoned player to have difficulty in merely hitting a ball.

In social learning, it is postulated that people tend to imitate (model) behavior they observe other persons emitting, particularly if it appears to result in the obtaining of a reinforcer. Hence, the more frequently an individual observes other persons displaying certain behaviors and obtaining rewards for doing so, the more likely it is that (s)he will also begin to behave in a similar manner. If an individual observes others making fun of another person and enjoying a mutual camaraderie in doing so, s(he) too will tend to join in. If, on the other hand, it is observed that people who talk loudly are asked to leave the room, the observer will tend to speak quietly and avoid being punished in a similar manner. When a person receives reinforcers for emitting a behavior that they have seen modeled, that behavior becomes an increasingly stronger component in the individual's repertoire, as one might expect.

Behavior therapy and behavioral counseling are based on these three types of learning. The goals are to teach people to make more appropriate and adaptive responses to environmental stimuli, to have people experience reinforcers for behaving appropriately and adaptively, and to provide good models of behavior to emulate.

Behavioral Counseling Techniques

There are a number of specific techniques behavior therapists utilize in helping clients to learn new skills and to experience more success in the tasks of daily living. These techniques include:

1. Behavioral assessment—pinpointing specific problems in operational terms and determining the strength of the problem behavior (i.e., how frequently or with what intensity it occurs) and what the conditions are that elicit and maintain (reinforce) the problem behavior.

2. Goal-setting—determining and stating specific objectives toward which the client will work in treatment.

3. Instructions—giving the client specific directions, prompts, cues, etc., that will induce a change in behavior.

4. Reinforcing and punishing—providing positive feedback for engaging in appropriate or adaptive behavior and negative feedback for engaging in inappropriate or maladaptive behavior.

5. Shaping—providing positive consequences for each successful successive step toward a therapeutic goal.

6. Modeling—demonstrating appropriate or adaptive behavior for the client to emulate.

7. Rehearsal—having the client practice new, appropriate, and adaptive behavior under the supervision of the therapist.

Additionally, more complex methodologies such as credit-incentive (token economy) systems, contingency (behavioral) contracting, assertive (personal effectiveness) training, etc., may also be employed in the course of behavioral counseling or behavior therapy. In all cases, the behavioral approach begins with a specification of the problem in which behavioral excesses and deficits are identified together with a functional analysis of their causes and effects. Goals, in terms of particular behaviors to be acquired and strengthened, or weakened and extinguished, are set. Then the client engages in a learning process designed to assist in the realization of the goals. In the learning process, the client practices new skills and is given a great deal of positive feedback for all progress made. The client's progress in learning and maintaining new skills is systematically evaluated at each step in the therapy program. When goals are reached, therapy may be terminated or new goals may be set and the whole process may be repeated until they too, are achieved.

Case Example

The following is an example of a behavioral counseling procedure, as recounted by a behavior therapist:

Alice P. Alice P. was an unmarried 67-year-old woman who had voluntarily sought out treatment at the local community mental health center. Everyone including Alice agreed that she was depressed. When I first met her, Alice was sitting by herself in a corner of the large activity room in the partial hospitalization (day treatment) unit. She seemed to be spending an inordinate amount of time staring dejectedly at the floor, while everyone else was engaged in some task or conversation. In a brief time, I was to lead a behaviorally based communications skills group in which Alice was scheduled to participate. I approached Alice, introduced myself, and attempted to engage her in a brief conversation about the program at the mental health center. I was a bit surprised to find that she was not at all hesitant to talk, was very friendly, and seemed to be in good control of herself.

After a few minutes of innocuous talk, I asked her why she had come to the mental health center. The bright, alert, and self-possessed person I'd just been chatting with disappeared and the picture of depression I'd seen earlier reappeared. Alice mumbled something about being completely inadequate. When pressed further, she explained that she did not see herself as a very good or competent person, that she had poor judgment, and that she felt she would never amount to anything. She figured she ought to do something about these feelings of poor self-worth and had come to the mental health center for help after she had started to consider suicide.

I asked her to tell me about the last time she felt inadequate. Alice told me that, just a few days ago, her mother had embarrassed her in front of several other people by going into a long-winded harangue about what a poor housekeeper she was. I asked if this sort of thing occurred often. Alice replied that her mother, who was 86 and lived in a retirement home a few blocks away, was always belittling her and had been since she was a teenager. Alice could never do anything right as far as her mother was concerned. When her mother criticized her in front of others, which was becoming more frequent, Alice found this especially upsetting. Yet, she hastened to tell me, she loved her mother dearly and her mother was really a wonderful person except for the fault-finding.

I asked Alice what one thing she would like to change about her relationship with her mother. She replied that she would certainly like to have her mother stop nagging her all the time, especially in public. I asked if she'd ever spoken to her mother about this problem. She had not. Alice claimed that she had tried, on many occasions, but had never quite been able to say what she was thinking. She was afraid. I asked if she would like to be able to confront her mother directly, the next time she was criticized. Alice replied that, for 40 years, there'd been nothing she wanted more. I suggested that we could, perhaps, work on this problem in the group. She hesitantly agreed that we might.

When it came time for Alice to work on her problem in the group, I asked her to choose another group member who could role-play her mother. Alice chose a middle-aged lady sitting next to her, with whom she appeared to be friendly. I asked her to explain to her "mother" what her mother was to say and do in order to approximate the incident that had occurred a few days ago. In a very subdued voice, she did so. We then played the scene through. The "mother" criticized and Alice just stood there, chin quivering, and took it. That was, according to Alice, just the way it went.

I suggested to Alice that we play the scene through again, and, this time, she was to interrupt her mother by saying "Mother, please stop criticizing me." Could she just say that, I asked? Alice thought she could. But, when we played the scene through again, Alice just stood there as before, only this time tears started to well up in her eyes. I stopped the action before they started to flow.

"I can't do it," she mumbled, "I can't look at her and say it."

"How about on the telephone?" suggested another member of the group, taking her literally. We all figured it was worth a try, so Alice and her "mother" sat back to back holding imaginary receivers to their ears. Her "mother" started criticizing and Alice just sat there. I went over to Alice, crouched down, and put an arm around her. She was shaking. I whispered in her ear, "Say 'Mother, stop it.' "

"I can't," she whispered.

"You can," I whispered, and repeated "Mother, stop it."

"Mother, stop it," she whispered.

"Louder," I prompted.

"Mother, stop it," said Alice. The torrent of criticism behind us stopped.

"Terrific!" I exclaimed as everyone in the group applauded. Alice started to cry, but she was smiling.

We tried it again and again, until Alice could interrupt her "mother" without being prompted. Then, we started to add more to Alice's statement "Mother, stop it. When you criticize me, you make me feel bad. I love you very much, but it's hard to be with you or talk with you when you criticize me. Would you please try to stop?" We practiced a few more times, and each time Alice seemed to get slightly less hesitant and became more confident.

The next day, Alice came up to me in the hallway, "I did it," she said.

"What?" I asked.

"I talked to Mother on the telephone last night, and when she started to criticize me, I did exactly what we practiced in the group yesterday."

"What happened?" I queried.

"She apologized!" exclaimed Alice. "She said she'd try to stop nagging me, and that if she starts again, I should just tell her to shut up!"

Commentary. This example of behavioral counseling illustrates the application of several specific procedures. It begins with targeting and pinpointing a specific problem in operational terms: Alice's inability to ask her mother to refrain from criticizing her. Then, an analysis of Alice's current level of skills is made: she demonstrates for the therapist exactly how she behaves in the problem situation. The procedure then entails a segment of training, in which Alice learns new skills. In the training segment, she is coached, prompted, and reinforced by the therapist. Additionally, she receives reinforcement from the treatment group (applause) when she finally masters the new skills. These new skills, finally, are applied in a real-life situation and result in a new and positive experience for Alice.

In behavioral counseling, the focus was not on Alice's depression per se, but rather on one specific difficulty in living that may have been contributing to the depressed state. Subsequent counseling (training) sessions would then focus on other specific situations or personal attributes which potentially lead to Alice's experience of failure, inadequacy, and distress, and she would be retrained to respond differently in each specific instance. In this manner, step by step, Alice would learn to become a more competent person and begin to experience herself as being capable of dealing more effectively with problems in daily living. With this restructuring of her behavior, Alice would begin to experience changes in feelings as well. As her repertoire of skills increases, her depressed feelings will concomitantly decrease.

Psychotherapy for the Aging: The Failure to Keep Pace

Recently there has been increased interest in adult development and aging, both on a scientific and a popular level. This interest has been generously (when compared with other areas) supported by the federal government, both in terms of funds available for research and demonstration grants and in the creation of agencies and institutes dealing specifically with the phenomena and problems of aging. As a result, a large body of knowledge has accumulated in this general area (Eisdorfer and Lawton, 1973; Schaie and Griffin, 1975).

In examining the scientific and professional literature, one finds that studies have focused predominantly on the basic *processes* of adult development and aging (i.e., changes in the nervous system, changes in cognitive abilities, changes in perception, etc.). Very few attempts to apply existing scientific knowledge in a therapeutic manner to the unique problems of the older person have been reported. Only recently has the attention of counselors and therapists been brought to bear on the mental health needs of older persons (Blake, 1975; Pressey, 1973; Pressey and Pressey, 1972). But even this heightened consciousness has not yet resulted in the development of many treatment innovations.

Prior to 1930, geriatric patients in mental hospitals received custodial care only (Wolff, 1956). Treatment of the geriatric patient has changed over the years, however, and currently there are somatic, milieu, and limited psychotherapeutic treatments available.

Somatic treatments, which include general physical care, medication, and electroshock, have been by far the most extensively used. Most institutions are designed primarily for physical care and tend, by their very nature, to center the residents' activities around bodily functioning. Psychopharmacological treatment, since the introduction of the ataractics, antidepressants, and psychomotor stimulants in the 1950s, has been the most prevalent of the somatic treatment methods used with geriatric patients, as it has been with younger patients as well.

Milieu therapy, which involves occupational and recreational therapy programs, attempts to construct a pleasant, cheerful, and optimistic environment and has been used with some success. Many older persons refuse, however, to participate in the planned activities, preferring simply to sit all day and not interact with either the staff or other residents (Paul, 1969).

Clinicians, apparently, are quite reluctant to conduct traditional psychotherapy with the older person. One reason is that many clinicians feel that older patients will not live "long enough" to repay their therapeutic "investment" in them. As older patients frequently are more reluctant to enter enthusiastically into the therapeutic process, may require more support throughout treatment, and may show slower and less dramatic gains in treatment, they may come to be seen as "low status" patients, requiring "second rate" therapy. Their problems, additionally, may not be particularly interesting to the therapist. "Thus, to conduct psychotherapy with an aged person is to enter a relationship with a low-status individual and to employ a technique that carries a low-status connotation with respect to its challenges to professional skill" (Kastenbaum, 1964, pp. 139–140). It has been pointed out that older patients may remind the therapist of his own mortality or conflicts with his own parents, issues that many would rather avoid. Additionally, there is a widespread belief that problems manifested by the aged are due to organic brain disease and, hence, are not really responsive to psychotherapy. Colleagues are frequently nonsupportive of those who choose to treat the elderly and have been heard to comment that such therapists must have a morbid preoccupation with death. Moreover, the clinician must confront the current cultural insensitivity and general lack of social responsiveness where problems of the aged are concerned. Thus, ageism, too, takes its toll (Cohen, 1976).

Because of this reluctance on the part of therapists to enter into therapeutic relationships with the aged, and the reluctance of older people to enter into therapy of any kind with anyone, relatively few elderly persons eventually receive psychotherapeutic services.

Encouraging Trends

In a departure from the traditional model, Linden (1953) reported some encouraging results utilizing group psychotherapy with older persons. However, applications of group methods have not been particularly widespread. It is a fairly common belief that group methods are not especially effective or efficient with older persons. When group psychotherapy has been attempted with the elderly, one of the usual criteria for selecting group members has been that they must be verbal and sufficiently mentally alert to follow and actively participate in group discussions. A large segment of institutionalized older persons, thus, are automatically eliminated from group therapies, since many do not display this ability and interest. Linden (1953) established selection criteria for his group as expressed desire to join the group, appearance of relative alertness, demonstration of at least a minimal range of affect, and a willingness to participate. Therefore, it seems reasonable to postulate that what success he noted may have, to some degree, been due to selection factors. The typical situation for institutionalized aged people, then, remains one of social impoverishment and lack of activity, where the primary (and, perhaps, only) treatment received is strictly medical (nonpsychiatric).

Older persons residing in institutions for the elderly (geriatric patients) are usually chronically ill, physically weak or debilitated, and organically or functionally limited. Quite often, though, the most striking characteristic of the geriatric patient group is not physical or mental limitations, but extremely poor social functioning. The silence which exists in a typical geriatric ward bespeaks the withdrawn, isolated, inactive, and asocial behavior of many geriatric patients.

Lindsley (1964) has a more optimistic view regarding treatment of geriatric patients. He emphasized the need for designing *prosthetic* environments for older persons, in order to restore more competent and appropriate behaviors.

> To prolong health, physicians offer aging persons a wide range of physiological prosthetics from vitamins and hormones, to increased oxygen. . . . Beyond providing eyeglasses, hearing aids, dentures, cribs, and crutches, however, science has done little to modify the external mechanical social environments of the aged. The skills of current behavioral science, and operant conditioning in particular, can provide more than compound lenses, audio amplifiers, and mechanical restraint and support. Behavioral engineers can design prosthetic environments to support the aged as crutches support their weight [Lindsley, 1964, p. 42].

Most geriatric patients manifest a variety of maladaptive and inappropriate behaviors. If more than one of these were dealt with at one time, patients' overall level of coping would be improved more rapidly, ward personnel could be utilized more effectively, and the cost of treatment would be reduced. Some research, although inconclusive, seems to indicate that operant methods may have such generalized effects (Skinner, 1953; Tilton, 1956; King, Armitage, and Tilton, 1960; Ayllon and Houghton, 1956; Ferster and DeMyer, 1962; Azrin and Lindsley, 1962). Moreover, by acquiring one new skill, patients "learn how to learn" other skills (Harlow, 1949). Once a learning "set" has been acquired, additional behaviors may be learned with increasing ease and efficiency.

Swenson (1965, 1971), working with psychiatric geriatric patients in an institutional setting, found reliably greater group participation in experimental tasks under operant conditioning procedures than under other procedures, which involved random reinforcement or extinction and approximated usual ward conditions. This finding supported the hypothesis that increases in desirable motoric, verbal, and cooperative social behavior could be made by highly nonverbal, asocial, and inactive geriatric psychiatric patients through the use of operant conditioning procedures.

One interesting example taken from this study concerns a patient who demonstrated marked changes across many behaviors. Minimal changes began to occur in his ward behavior even during individual and cooperative conditioning periods, and then marked verbal and cooperative motor changes occurred during the cooperative plus verbal part of the experimental procedure. These changes occurred both in the experimental room and on the ward and continued throughout the study. When the marked changes began, the patient immediately received a considerable amount of social reinforcement from ward personnel and even from other patients. Reinforcement in the form of being allowed to smoke on the ward again with the other patients was also given him for his "good" behavior. The ward personnel were quite amazed by the general change in his behavior. His behavior in the experimental room was consistent with his behavior on the ward, at recreation, and at occupational therapy. He praised others for their activity and tried to encourage others to be active and sociable. Quite often, both in the experimental room and on the ward, he would say to the others, "What can I do now to earn a cigarette?" or, "What can I do to help you?" Eventually this kind of behavior became somewhat annoying to the ward personnel and patients, and medication was instituted!

Because only very limited psychotherapeutic practice is conducted with institutionalized geriatric patients (Kastenbaum, 1964), it is encouraging to find that such a relatively brief therapeutic effort as that employed by Swenson (1965, 1971), based on learning theory principles and techniques, was effective in an experimental situation in achieving desired motor, cooperative, and social behavior in institutionalized older persons. It seems probable, therefore, that a variety of appropriate behaviors could be instated and problem behaviors eliminated in geriatric patients through use of instruction, with reinforcement contingent upon desired behaviors.

It is proposed that therapeutic efforts with older persons might be more productive if they were directed toward specific behavioral deficits or excesses exhibited by individuals in their daily living situations. This would entail establishing individualized behavioral programs for each person receiving treatment. Such endeavors in institutional settings would probably require complete patient–staff–administration cooperation, as Ayllon (Mishler, 1964) achieved in his experimental ward of female psychotic patients. Such a program would, indeed, mandate consistent support and cooperation from all treatment personnel.

Geriatric institutions or wards tend to be quite large and understaffed. In such situations, there is little opportunity or time to pay attention to and systematically reinforce all desirable behavior. It may be likely that such large nonreinforcing or random-reinforcing units, in which passive, quiet, nondemanding, inactive behavior tends to be the norm (because it is reinforced), would have to be greatly restructured if behavior change is ever to occur.

The atrophy of social interaction and physical activity for older persons is neither a desirable nor a necessary phenomenon. The continued prevalence of such apathetic, unhappy, poorly motivated, and withdrawn behavior in the older person is conceivably due, in large part, to the generally rather unimaginative, superficial approaches taken by traditional medical and social gerontology, with emphasis primarily on physical care and psychopharmacological treatment. With such an emphasis, the emotional needs of the older person, his/her feelings of individuality, independence, and self-worth, self-reliance, and self-care are not stressed and eventually become diminished (Lipsett, 1969).

Our discussion, up to now, has centered upon the issues and examples of institutional care. This is so because the clinical literature has, historically, focused almost exclusively upon institutional care when discussing treatments for older persons. While this may, on the surface, seem rather narrow-minded of the professional community it is, in reality, an indication that the literature is well attuned to practice. Most older persons receive treatment in institutions, if they receive it at all. Relatively few are seen in the outpatient services of mental health centers, hospitals, clinics, and in private practice, for reasons discussed earlier. While this has, most definitely, been the case for some time, it is not necessarily good, desirable, or mandatory.

Behavioral approaches may be more conducive than many others in attracting older persons to services offered outside institutional contexts, as well as being relatively effective in meeting their needs. Groups in assertion and communication skills have, for example, experienced increasing numbers of older participants when offered in community settings. (For an in-depth view, see Chapter 1 in this volume, "Assertive Training Groups for the Aging," by Eugenie G. Wheeler.)

As has been pointed out, many older persons, especially those residing in institutions of various kinds, but even many living in the community, fail to engage in physical activity, verbal behavior, and cooperative social interaction with other residents, personnel, family, peers, and friends. From the behavioral point of view, such deficits would be considered to be the result of the person's immediate environment and reinforcement history. As Lindsley has said,

> In precise behavioral terms, this means either that the reinforcers currently programmed to his immediate environment are no longer adequate or that the old person has simply lost the ability to be reinforced. The difference is of great importance and should be tested experimentally by attempting to reinforce his/her behavior with a wide range of events [Lindsley, 1964, p. 51].

Lindsley concluded that if appropriate historical or expanded, immediate personal reinforcers could be located for each individual, newer and more generally available events (general conditioned reinforcers used in society) might even be conditioned to the idiosyncratic reinforcers, and that by gradual shaping and conditioning the older person could be given a new interest in contemporary life.

The behavioral approach offers an innovative and potentially powerful means of meeting the needs of older persons and caregivers, in both institutional and community settings. Its focus is on the specific, concrete, and situational, rather than the global, abstract, and generalized. It emphasizes learning new skills rather than rehashing old problems. It casts the therapist as an active agent of change, an educator, and a manager rather than a passive sounding-board or font of tea and sympathy. It views the client as a learner and as capable of taking immediate, positive action to reshape and improve the quality of his/her own life rather than as a helpless victim of circumstance who must come to accept his plight. It offers a nonstigmatizing, relatively inexpensive, simple, and flexible means for directly confronting problems in living that may be experienced by older persons. It offers the caregiver an empirically validated technology that is effective with a wide variety of problems, marketable, and amenable to evaluation.

Nontraditional Models of Service Delivery

A nontraditional approach to counseling and psychotherapy does not mandate a traditional model of service delivery. The behavioral approach is especially conducive to alternative modes of intervention. One example of such an alternative is the Expediter Project conducted in Tacoma, Washington (Wahler, Johnson, and Ulrich, 1972), which utilized nineteen indigenous paraprofessionals to provide assistance in living to persons recently released from a mental hospital.

> It is apparent that office- or institution-bound psychotherapy, casework, counseling, or supportive relationships are often not enough. When life is badly awry, people also need help with some or many aspects of their ecological milieu. In other words, they need someone to expedite—someone to provide information, to lend a hand when and where it is needed, and to intercede if need be. The office-bound professional has neither the time nor range of information to function as a situational therapist. This is true no matter how badly his client may need intercession, specific and applicable information, or a tangible helping hand. Thus, to translate the notion of "working with the total person" into functional reality, professionals with expertise in inside processes must have a team-mate who is expert in working with outside processes [Wahler, Johnson, and Ulrich, 1972. p. i, ii].

Those persons who received the expediter's services showed a lower rate of reinstitutionalization at a six-month follow-up than a matched control group which did not receive these services. The expediters did not directly or systematically attempt to modify the behavior of their clients, but behavior change occurred nonetheless. The expediter is a concept which potentially solves the problem of limited manpower to provide the consistent and integrated support necessary for the success of behavioral programs. With training and under the proper supervision, an expediter could become an integral part of a treatment team.

Perhaps one of the most significant current aims of the behavioral approach would be to explore and document the ability of older persons to work with their peers in a helping way, i.e., to be an expediter. In both the scientific literature and popular press, great emphasis has been placed in recent years on the effectiveness and efficiency of child, adolescent, and young adult peers serving as volunteers, paraprofessionals, lay peer counselors, or helpers. But apparently the significance of this work has not, until recently, been systematically utilized in attempts to discover or demonstrate similar beneficial helping relationships for older persons. (See Chapter 8 in this volume, "A Peer Counseling Program in Action," by Bratter and Tuvman, for a detailed example.) The behavioral approach seems well suited to explore and document the ability of older persons to work with their peers, to define certain roles such as that of the expediter, and to evaluate the outcomes of the peer counseling process for both the helpers and those receiving assistance.

It may well be that institutionalized residents of homes for the aged could carry out some of the activities and duties which are currently being performed only by paid employees of the institution. By allowing residents to carry out many of the helping and other kinds of duties, current staff could be freed to spend more time with the residents who would benefit from more intensive professional care and attention. The opportunity, indeed the necessity, for the aged resident to contribute to his own self-care, assist in the care of his less able peers, and perform the various chores that are necessary to the ongoing processes of his aged community would be generated by a value system that expects and therefore rewards such productive action. It is anticipated that great personal satisfaction will be realized by the individuals of the community in the enhancement of their self-worth as a result of the performance of useful acts—work as opposed to hobby and craft activities alone. This same approach could be attempted, as well, in the community with "well" older persons assisting in the care and support of their "less well" or "infirm" peers.

Another nontraditional model of service delivery which has effectively used behavioral approaches to treatment was pioneered by the Tri-Counties Regional Center for the Developmentally Disabled in Santa Barbara, California (Swenson and Rosenstein, 1978).

The center provides diagnostic evaluation, counseling, and lifelong planning services for the developmentally disabled and their families. A nonprofit organization, it has a board of directors composed of parents, professionals, and community leaders. It secures funds by contracts with the California Department of Health to provide mental health services in three counties.

The center thus acts as a broker for purchase of services from independent professionals in the community. The professional is accountable to the regional center for the quality of the service. The center is accountable to the state for the availability of service to those in need. The state is accountable to the taxpayers for the proper disbursement of public funds designated for this purpose.

Through this model of service delivery, the center mobilizes and makes efficient use of resources in the community to provide services for its developmentally disabled clients. Thus, public health care is provided on a large scale and integrated effectively without duplication of the services available in the private sector.

In providing psychological services to Regional Center clients, the agency issues contracts to professional, licensed psychologists in the community. These contracts specify the clients to be served, the precise nature of the problems to be remediated, the period during which services are authorized, the behavioral objectives toward which the client is to work, and the reimbursement for the services to be provided.

These professionals each maintain a staff of highly trained paraprofessionals called "behavior analysts" (after Tharp and Wetzel, 1969). The behavior analysts, under the supervision of the psychologist, design behavioral programs tailored to the needs of each particular client and then work with the clients, their families, teachers, and other caregivers *in the communities where the clients live* to assist the clients in reaching their behavioral objectives. The procedures utilized are based on operant conditioning, classical conditioning, and social learning, and the behavior analyst functions as trainer, consultant, and evaluator.

This model of service delivery could easily be adopted for working with older persons. Its strengths are that high-quality services are provided at home and in the community. They are provided directly by a trained person who does not carry the label "psychotherapist," and they are provided inexpensively. Again, this model offers a way to combat the shortage of caregivers and nonstigmatizing resources available to older persons and also offers a mechanism to involve older persons with their peers: the elderly themselves can be trained in behavioral methods and become behavior analysts.

Pressey (1973) identifies older and retired professionals as probably the most effective corps of counselors for the elderly because of their training, their interest in older people, and the likelihood that they would be living with the people they would be serving. These are still trained professionals, however, and not simply older persons learning how to care for other elderly persons. Such a group would be comparatively small or, at least, not numerous enough to carry out all the needed services or care for the rapidly growing older population. Perhaps persons from this professional group could, however, serve as instructors and/or supervisors for other older persons serving as peer helpers (expediters or behavior analysts).

Behavioral approaches are not, most certainly, a panacea for all problems of older persons and their caregivers. They do, however, offer a viable alternative that deserves the serious consideration of those who are concerned with the welfare of the constantly growing aged segment of the population.

Kassabaum (1969) states that

> . . . uselessness, boredom, and fear of sickness and death are some of the older person's greatest difficulties, and . . . to be allowed to putter in a garden or play shuffleboard is not a satisfactory substitute for more meaningful activity. . . . No two older people are alike, and about all we can be sure of is that there is at least one factor in common, and that is their desire to live their lives with as much freedom as their condition justifies [Kassabaum, 1969, pp. 2, 6].

Behavioral approaches offer the means to achieve this freedom. With the proper and creative use of behavioral technology and the development of new roles for older persons in its implementation, we can change the prospects for those of us who are destined to live our later years dependent, restricted, and unhappy in "... gilded cages where domesticated canaries are happy but eagles with clipped wings suffer the torment of the damned " (Harrison, 1970, p. 3).

Recommended Readings

Bandura, A. *Principles of behavior modification.* New York: Holt, Rinehart and Winston, 1969.

Reese, E. P. *Human behavior: analysis and application.* Dubuque, Iowa: Brown, 1978.

Schwitzgebel, R. K. and Kolb, D. A. *Changing human behavior.* New York: McGraw-Hill, 1974.

12

The Approach of Pastoral Psychology

John M. Vayhinger

"Pastoral psychology" is not a distinctive theoretical or technical approach to counseling and therapy comparable, say, to psychoanalysis or behavioral psychology, which have fairly well-defined procedures. It depends for its effectiveness, especially with older people, upon the existence of deep trust and good rapport with the minister, priest, or rabbi. It is aided by an atmosphere of moral and spiritual concern and by the parishioners' understanding that the pastor is primarily concerned with their salvation. It is often facilitated by the nature of the problem—e.g., religious conflict or the fear of dying. The development of pastoral psychology shows its particular relevance for the elderly.

Over the past couple of hundred years there have been striking changes in the relation between church and state, with government gradually taking over many functions formerly performed by religious institutions. One area where the changes have been less noticeable is that of the aging, where church and synagogue still share much of the concern for and care of older persons. The involvement of the aging with religion is far greater than their participation in any other social institution. (This includes both their Sunday church attendance and many church-related activities during the week.) Visitations during hospitalization and final illness and the performing of funerals is almost exclusively the task of the clergy.

Pastoral counseling has been part of the clergyman's work for several centuries; how then can it be considered "nontraditional"? Perhaps the answer is that it has been treated as a purely religious matter or just as a helpful ancillary procedure. Only recently has it been accepted by psychiatric and psychological professionals as a legitimate and effective therapeutic medium. By now it is apparent that the pastoral approach is often advantageous with older people because they do not resist counseling from the minister or rabbi; in fact, they expect it! And as the clergy have become better trained in therapeutic techniques, they are increasingly able to function like other nontraditional therapists in helping distressed, timorous, and resistant older people.

Church and Clergy: Resource for the Elderly

Many "grandpersons" turn to religion with renewed fervor.[1] Perhaps part of the motivation stems from the numerous problems which face older people in any society, because of the gradual approach of the dying experience, because they have more time to think about the meaning of life than before, and perhaps because they are "wiser" than when the enthusiasm of youth interfered with reasoning and judicious observation. Certainly, the more years we've lived, the greater the experience we've had in which to reflect, the greater the hunger to explain ourselves to ourselves, and the deeper the need to justify our existence on this earth. Thus, many elderly persons turn to the churches and synagogues and religious experience, as may be seen on any Friday evening or Sunday morning in our religious houses.

Religious activities do not decline as much with disabilities in old age as other social and professional activities do. In fact, in one Kansas study, church was found to be so important that "... regularity of attendance seemed to be an index of the measure of the man" (Twente, 1970, p. 24). Another study in Wake County, North Carolina, found that there were 149 memberships in religious groups for every 100 older persons, but only 38 memberships in all of the other community institutions and organizations taken together (Phil-

[1]There are many names to indicate those persons reaching old age, and one designation this writer finds interesting is "grandperson." If we have *grand*sons and *grand*daughters, then it follows we may call the seniors *grand*parents and *grand*persons. While not popular yet, it does reflect the respect in which grandpersons are held in churches and synagogues.

blad and Rosencranz, 1969). Though wide variations occur within and between differing social groups, studies have consistently revealed, especially in smaller communities and away from the largest urban centers, that nine out of every ten persons aged 60 and older participated in some way in churches and synagogues.

Thus, it seems appropriate that any study of newer treatment of older persons would include, if not begin in, the institution where the greatest participation already exists.

Churches and synagogues, being family oriented, have always been concerned about the health and welfare of their older members. Historically, age was a prime consideration for wisdom, so that the elders of the tribe or society were usually given honor and respect. A basic standard of the New Testament is, "If anyone does not provide for his relatives, and especially for his own family, he has disowned the faith and is worse than an unbeliever" (I Timothy 5:8).

The responsibility of the church to care for its elderly and the importance of religion to the elderly underlies the help they receive. One study done in Minnesota indicates that more than half the men and almost 70 percent of the women regarded religion as the most important thing in their lives. It revealed that "a sense of serenity and decreased fear of death tended to accompany conservative religious beliefs which stress the reality of the afterlife," though not necessarily removing all anxiety concerning the stresses of dying (Stotsky, 1968, p. 31). The study also showed that the clergies aid patients greatly and strongly reinforce the psychiatrist's efforts, helping to counteract boredom, loneliness, and feelings of rootlessness and alienation. Religious belief in existence after death challenges patients to perform purposeful, preparatory rituals, and to remain occupied so they do not have to wrestle with the doubt and anguish of the emptiness facing them (Stotsky, 1968, pp. 122, 123, 133).

Another piece of research revealed that while attendance in a house of worship does not increase steadily with age, *the importance attached to religion in people's lives does.* Seventy-one percent of the public 65 and over feels religion is very important in their own lives, compared with only 49 percent of those under 65. Fewer of the older group identify their religion as "none" than do the younger public (Gross et al., 1978, p. 105).

Certainly, increasing incidence of mortality among loved ones and friends focuses the attention of older persons on their own deprivation, grief, and isolation. Furthermore, the older citizen looks for religious emotional support for experiences of bereavement, illness, social deprivation, and other personal and social problems and shows increasing preoccupation with philosophic values and religious ideas (Gray and Moberg, 1977, p. 65).

The Goals of Pastoral Psychology

With their background of involvement in religion and participation in church activities, the elderly naturally turn to the clergy in time of crisis. Studies have revealed that more people turn to their ministers and rabbis in an emergency, especially an emotional crisis, than to any other professional group. Like other professionals, some clergy may suffer from "gerontophobia," but in general they are the closest to older persons, on deeper social and personal levels, and have been so for longer periods of time. And most clergy see pastoral caring or counseling as a crucial part of their function.

What is the goal of pastoral therapy? Let's call it *spiritual well-being,* which is defined by the 1975 National Interfaith Coalition on Aging as "the affirmation of life in a relationship with God, self, community, and environment that nurtures and celebrates wholeness." *Spiritual* permeates and gives meaning to all life; it affirms our dependence on the source of life, God the Creator. *Spiritual well-being* indicates wholeness in contrast to fragmentation and isolation; it is rooted in a community of faith in which "one grows to accept the past, to be aware and alive in the present and to live in hope of fulfillment" (Gray and Moberg, 1977, pp. 202–203). The Church would, of course, speak of "salvation" and "holiness" rather than "therapy" and "adjustment." Though certainly not equivalents, they do carry considerable similarity in goal definition.

Goals for the pastoral counselor working with older persons have been specified as: (1) to help lift up the dignity and worth of each individual, and (2) to enable the aging as children of God to maintain their pride, self-respect, and self-esteem so that they may continue as productive, creative human beings within the framework of their potential (Clingan, 1975). Since these goals are obviously similar to those of psychotherapy with older persons, pastor and psychotherapist and the elderly will benefit when all three cooperate in planning and working together (see Young and Meiburg, 1960).

Jewish and Christian views of the elderly are similar. In Ecclesiastes 8:7 both Christians and Jews are taught to "despise not a man in his old age," and in Exodus 20:12 "honor your father and your mother." Jesus taught his followers to minister to the hungry, thirsty, sick, imprisoned, poor, and widowed (in Matthew 25:31–40), which covers the needs of many elderly. According to the rabbis, oldness is not of itself a virtue; only wisdom and knowledge of the Torah determine the value of old age. The rabbis teach that the truly effective life is one that goes on growing and developing to the very end of living and which culminates, like Moses at age 120, in the person living to his or her very last day with full physical and mental powers and relationships. This kind of instruction certainly influences the older person with religious faith to seek help, including preventive or remedial psychotherapy, when needed.

The Pastoral Counselor at Work

I am an ordained minister in good standing in the United Methodist Church (New York Conference), a licensed clinical psychologist with a practice, and a graduate school professor. I have sought to combine in my vocation that spiritual direction and concern with secular professional skills, cooperating with private and governmental institutions, so that the preferred way to care for the needs of older persons may be found.

Sometimes my pastoral therapy is very similar to the clinical procedures which are followed by many clinical psychologists and psychiatrists. Take the case of Nancy, for instance.

Case Example

Nancy. Nancy is 77 at the time of this writing. A widow for four years, she was referred to me when her depression and profound sense of guilt did not yield to her physician's medications. At first she felt guilty and self-condemning because she had denied a desired form of sex to her husband when he was alive and then had responded angrily to his querulousness during his last illness. She had become fed up with his constant demands and sarcasm and responded to him with hostility. He had a final fatal coronary just a few minutes after her angry words. Her questions as to the therapist's "being a Christian," were simply answered affirmatively, and almost immediately trust was established in the therapeutic relationship. Her sensorium was intact, her thought patterns were logical and reality-oriented, and her contact with reality was adequate.

Exploration of the patient's early life uncovered a compulsive, controlling, belittling mother of very real ability and skills, a favored younger sister, a father who traveled and was gone for long periods, to the mother's chagrin. The psychiatric depression extended back into grade school with varying episodes, though no hospitalizations. A major factor in her dynamics was rooted in a profound feeling of inadequacy, of being unloved and being rejected by everyone, including her own only child, a daughter, who cared for her mother with angry reluctance but considerable efficiency.

The major components of the depression were the intense anger generated by the degrading by the mother and husband—turned inward toward the self—the loss of ability to do much more than care for her small three-room house, and the disrupted relationship with the daughter.

The therapy included two main areas: (1) exploring and aerating early felt failures with resulting emotional reevaluation and relief from self-condemnation for the past and, most important, a recovery of a belief in a loving God who could give support and comfort through the aches and pains of old age and the approaching dying experience, and (2) a redirecting and sublimating of the energy being used in anger, making possible a lifting of the depression for longer and longer periods until the patient could live a more active life consistent with her frailty and her arthritis. A most important part of the reconstructive therapy was involvement with her pastor and the church congregation and the specifically Methodist belief system she was able to depend upon through her reinvolvement with the church. Now the depressive periods are quite short and do not overwhelm her as before. She is able to do work consistent with her age, and the relationship with the daughter and her family has improved very much.

Of course, many clergymen have not had training in theological school that would enable them to deal directly with the problems of severely distressed older persons. A survey of more than a hundred members of the clergy in a large Midwestern city revealed that only 29 percent had had preparation to help them understand the experiences and feelings of people as they grow older, and still fewer felt the preparation was adequate (Moberg, 1975).

But there are things any minister, priest, or rabbi can do, no matter how meager his training in therapy and counseling. Since he has the trust of the members of his congregation and good rapport with them, he is in a favored position to give some kind of help, not only for religious problems but for almost any concern about which they come to talk with him. He can listen, encouraging the person to present the problem as clearly as possible. He can accept the expression of feeling, realizing this has cathartic value. He can pray with the person. He may be able honestly to offer reassurance and to help him or her formulate goals and plan steps for their attainment. If he senses that the person is basically confused or upset, or so ill as to need expert help, he is in the best position to make referral to a psychiatrist, a clinical psychologist, a psychiatric social worker, or a community mental health center. It is very important, of course, for the minister/rabbi to be well aware of the mental health resources in his community.

Counseling and Reassuring the Dying

One problem area is particularly appropriate for the minister, priest, or rabbi: distress centering on the fear of death. Aiding and comforting dying persons, though somewhat new to psychiatric and psychological therapists, has long been a part of every pastor's daily task.

In the same way that good personal adjustment and active religious involvement are correlated, so does a person's attitude toward death make a great difference in his or her behavior. "Believers" often feel a greater sense of usefulness, may engage in prayer for each other, may act to find forgiveness for sins, which relieves a sense of guilt, and may discover that suffering has meaning and value for deepening one's awareness of self in sensing a meaning to life (Gray and Moberg, 1977).

Nonbelievers are more likely to realize death is approaching, which may be a disturbing thought (at least subconsciously) and, for those without belief in life eternal, very anxiety-arousing. Nonbelievers may also be bothered by feelings of guilt, even while saying they do not believe in sin, and may find it more difficult to believe there is dependable order or meaning in a universe with a Creator and Sustainer (Gray and Moberg, 1977, p. 85. Illustrative case histories follow p. 101).

A few years ago, Elisabeth Kübler-Ross reported in a NIMH Workshop on Mental Health for Clergy at the Anderson School of Theology that when she was in a terminal psychiatric ward in Chicago, she could see little difference between terminal cancer patients who were religious and those who were not in their attitudes toward dying and in the process of dying. But, she added, when she was transferred to a unit where terminal patients were not psychiatrically confused, she found a great difference in the dignity, acceptance, and other attitudes in the dying patient between the religious and the nonreligious, with the religious persons showing greater acceptance and inner peace, and needing less medication for pain.

Death attitudes are complex, depending upon the depth and intensity of the particular beliefs of the persons involved; the person may feel "forgiven" or "saved" or "close to God," may be aware of approaching death, may feel supported by the presence of the clergy and family, etc. But it is my experience that most persons who believe sincerely that death brings reunion with loved ones approach death differently from those who believe that death brings only nothingness and the end of all consciousness. A spiritual leader is in a unique position to help one face death in a religious way. The clergy person is indeed

> a symbol and a substitute; he must also be a listener. Where both respect and trust can be established, a person often pours out all kinds of festering matter: remembrance, regrets, gratitude and guilt. A free form of confessional is a necessary self-purging. Often, people reorder their own feelings and have resources where they become their own therapists [Moriarty, 1967, pp. 187–188].

A minister can be a compassionate, understanding, tolerant, and forgiving representative of Jesus Christ, guiding the person toward spiritual wholeness and salvation.

For many, says Lazar D. Brener, "religion puts together some of the puzzle of life and death." The religious community should have the same attitude toward the elderly in retirement centers and nursing homes as they have to members of their constituency, both the well and the sick. It is certainly therapeutic to the residents of these facilities when the clergy and congregations can provide compassion, understanding, and a sense of dignity. "Though we may talk about dying with dignity," concludes Brener, "the emphasis should be on *living with dignity.* Living involves hope and optimism." With the aid of spiritual reinforcement (or we could read "therapy") and the serenity that accompanies religious convictions, "the older person is better able to accept the ills and limitations that may befall him in old age" (Brener, quoted in Clingan, 1975, pp. 44–45).

Community as a Form of Therapy

Still another resource in religious groups comes from their being a community, which is a primary goal of any church or synagogue, and which is also a very old form of therapy. Not only is man a communitarian being, but "God is not a lonely person; rather, there is a community within the very being of God. The supreme divine community within is the ultimate model of all forms of community" (Deeken, 1972, p. 95).

It is a well-known fact that older people have a psychological need to feel useful and wanted. Especially living in a mass society, older persons often underestimate their own importance, and it is in the daily functions of the congregation that many find their advice, presence, and talents sought and appreciated. New and old forms of volunteer and official service in the congregation provide a form of behavior therapy in a different setting. While group therapy and psychodrama have developed on the edge of the religious communities, the church and synagogue are still, in my opinion, the site of the largest number of dynamic and therapeutic groups.

This discussion leads naturally to the use of religious institutions as *natural treatment centers* as well as sources for referral to psychotherapy. The Harris poll reported in November 1974 that 75 percent of seniors would prefer to spend most of their time with people of all ages, and that 22 percent already gave themselves in unpaid volunteer work in settings such as churches. This suggests that grandpersons in our society form a vast untapped pool of energy for paraprofessional therapy when recruited and trained by professional therapists, as is shown by the many peer counseling programs for older people (see Part II of this volume). Religious leaders trained in psychotherapy can in turn train some of the older members of our churches and synagogues with the goal of providing assistance to mental health centers and mental hospitals.

Of course ministers and lay therapists must first be freed from the influence of many myths and stereotypes about aging, so they can in turn help others to free themselves. James A. Peterson, an ordained clergyman who is Professor of Sociology at the University of Southern California, lists six myths of aging which he feels the churches/synagogues can aid in eradicating (see Clingan, 1975):

1. *The rocking chair myth* that grandpersons want only to retire and loaf, which is accurate only when society insists that they are useless. "The church/synagogue needs to affirm that God has a place for all persons to give themselves, regardless of age."

2. The myth that *older persons are physically incapacitated* has to yield to facts. Ninety percent of persons over 65 are mobile, 8 percent need help in getting around, and only 1 or 2 percent are institutionalized because of their immobility. Many simply need exercise in order to be able to function.

3. The *myth of the senile mind.* Vocabulary and conceptualization may actually improve in aging persons, whose thinking often is slower, but whose brain functions are usually intact. Pseudo-senility is more likely to come about through lack of attention than through physical atrophy.

4. Another myth is that *grandpersons are useless and want to be "disengaged."* Although they sometimes need transportation, we should remember that we have had superior professors who taught into their 80s, doctors who practiced well into their 70s, parents who kept involved with their families through the 80s and into the 90s. This writer has a mother living in his family who is 85, and parents-in-law 85 and 89 still in their own home just around the corner. Disengagements are more likely to happen when society or younger persons withdraw from the grandpersons.

5. A fifth myth, i.e., *constant depression is typical of older persons,* is refuted by the discovery that most citizens over age 65 are no more depressed than those under 65, though they do suffer many periods of grief due to the loss of relatives and friends.

6. The last myth is that *older persons are not capable of participating in and are not interested in public affairs.* One has only to look at the Congress and Supreme Court of the United States, or the premiers of many countries, or the presidents of large companies to realize this is not so. Churches look to the aging for leadership; pastors, bishops, nuns, popes, and other religious officials continue to function well past the 65-year deadline customary in industry, education, and other secular institutions.

The church/synagogue can and often does take the lead in attacking and counteracting these harmful myths and stereotypes. This is an essential first step in mobilizing an army of volunteers and friendly visitors, whose humanizing and therapeutic influence can be tremendous.

For the 1971 White House Conference on Aging, David O. Moberg identified six areas of "spiritual need": (1) sociocultural needs, (2) relief from anxieties and fears, (3) preparation for death, (4) personality integration, (5) freedom from personal disunity, and (6) a philosophy of life (see McClellan, 1977). He may well be thinking of these as psychological needs demanding new types of therapy as he issues this challenge to the religious communities:

> If our religious institutions do not actively and specifically take on the spiritual needs of mankind as a primary responsibility, it may well be that no other institution in society will. After all, there is only one thing

> that churches and other religious bodies can do best. That one thing is to accentuate the spiritual well-being of the elderly lest it be overlooked completely. Man is a spiritual being and therefore cannot live by bread alone [Moberg, 1973].

Lazar D. Brener, Executive Director of Hooverwood, Indianapolis Jewish Home, Inc., insists that one of the fresh forms of therapy in the next decade will occur in nursing homes, health care centers, and nursing centers. Such counseling will cover: (1) the decision to enter such facilities, and (2) treatment of the traumatic experience when independence is lost, along with the sense of worth, to be replaced by a feeling of rejection by relatives and friends. Intermittent treatment by rabbis, pastors, or priests renders continuous spiritual support through visitation, and clergy on the staff may offer pastoral counseling since the clergy would be part of the professional team that provides total care. "There is," he insists,

> no substitute for a personal call by the pastor, priest, or rabbi, or a congregational member who shows loving concern. For residents who cannot continue to attend the church/synagogue, religious services must be provided for them in the facility. Here, clergy and congregations can be of great assistance. It will meet the spiritual needs of many. Also, it has been observed that even for the brain damaged, senile, or confused resident, religious services may bring to them some modicum of serenity, and also may return them temporarily to the world of reality. The prayers acquired as a youngster may still be remembered by the confused elderly [Brener, quoted in McClellan, 1977, p. 44].

There are many unique opportunities that congregations may seize in ministering to grandpersons. Since a religious congregation is: (1) a volunteer group with no power to demand participation except the call of faith, (2) composed of a great number of older persons who can quite literally control its finances and direction, (3) an historical institution of the Judeo-Christian tradition surviving thousands of years with basically the same ingredients, (4) a social institution, (5) an institution which has a biblical/historical foundation based on a series of covenants with God, and (6) an institution which has the most potential economic power of any institution in existence, especially when seen in an interfaith context, ". . . *it has as its most important objective to give meaning and values to human life.*" (Clingan, 1975, pp. 27, 28).

One medical professor suggests that households with older members would find an advantage in

> starting each day with a devotional period when scripture, poetry, or inspirational literature is read aloud. Sometimes the grandperson can take charge of this interval, helping the family off to a good day's beginning. For those religiously inclined, prayers at some time during the day tend to reduce tensions [Poe, 1967, p. 40].

Poe also encourages elderly persons to keep up their interest in church activities. Though it may be bothersome to accompany them to their church/synagogue,

> the contact with the people there, the Mass or sermon, the quiet meditation, may be of vast importance to her well-being. . . . A church service or group meeting is an occasion for her to dress up—to fix her hair and wear something stylish—all therapeutic measures for a person who wants to keep on enjoying life [Poe, 1967, p. 18].

When older persons are sick, therapists may suggest a pastor's visit: "The old need to have their religious beliefs treated with respect," says Poe, especially by therapists who are attempting to help them overcome depression, loneliness, disorientation, and anxiety. "The spiritual needs of the old are not really different from those that we all have, but the feeling that death is near makes these needs more important. By honoring them, we can contribute much to an aging person's peace of mind" (Poe, 1967, pp. 18–19).

Religious Resources Available for Therapy

Some psychotherapists and writers on aging almost completely neglect the significance of religious beliefs and communities. For example, one otherwise well-researched and well-written book made only three brief references to religious data (Blau, 1973). Some books have no religious references at all. However, many if not most students of aging would agree that our civilization is based on the belief in God and, as Martin Buber said, "we have been brought up in His awareness and it would be a sad day if we miss it" (Maurus, 1976, p. 109).

A number of psychotherapists have been discovering the resources inherent in their patients' religious beliefs and in available religious institutions. Victor Frankl's "logotherapy," for one, stresses the importance of meaning and value in life and is sympathetic toward faith and religious belief (Frankl, 1955; Deeken, 1972). There seems to be an increasing openness on the part of therapists to respect and encourage the older person's religious beliefs with their implicit strength and goal orientation. Therapists with a personal faith and solid roots in the synagogue or church are uniting their therapeutic skills and personal participation with elderly grandpersons in church settings. Perhaps they are heeding Browning's famous invitation:

> Grow old along with me
> The best is yet to be.
> The last of life for which the first was made:
> Our times are in His hand
> Who saith, "A Whole I planned.
> Trust God, see all, nor be afraid."

In closing, let us look at the religious resources available for therapeutic use as described by Seward Hiltner and others in a summary of a 1974 workshop, "Toward a Theology of Aging."

Emphasizing the need to learn about older aging persons, Dr. Hiltner noted a "learning period," in which persons past 65 years of age continue to learn and grow. "There is," he writes, "an increase in vitality and in the capacity for work that can bring self-respect when older persons may continue to work in useful, positive positions, volunteer or paid for." In discussion groups, the members noted the importance of hope in the face of difficulties and suggested that "a realistic confrontation of death in both senses (as in Judaism and Christianity) combined with the faith that somehow (the way is not known to us) death is not the end," is the most basic difficulty that genuine hope must control.

One of Hiltner's discussion groups took the family (or household) of God metaphor of the Bible and suggested that recapturing its biblical intent, but putting into its concrete context the whole range of ages now familiar to us, could be of great value not only for the traditional purpose (as a model of the church) but also as a theological statement regarding all mankind in a heterogeneous society. With more people living longer and with at least more potential for creativity, the age span of the family of God must be considered in a new light.

Apparently, Dr. Hiltner is giving the therapist a model for treatment in which the goal is the religious concept of the common family of children (of God), approximating the therapeutic model of restoring or maturing the patient to a level of relationship, independence, and the ability to love and work.

We have seen that religious concepts and religious personnel constitute valuable therapy for grandpersons. After a number of years when psychotherapy (both psychiatric and psychological) has pretty well ignored religion, the 1980s promise to *recover* many of the concepts, a considerable number of institutions, and a great many of the professional personnel in churches and synagogues as an exciting and productive part of our responsibilities in the care and treatment of the older persons in our culture.

First, the seminaries are training the clergy in concepts and skills, not only in the *care* of older persons, but also in their *counseling.*

Second, a great many persons in the professional field of psychotherapy are becoming more open to religious ideas and to increasingly better-trained clergy as members of therapy teams.

Third, there are over 600 pastoral counseling centers in the United States, church based or independently organized, where persons over age 55 are seen for counseling.

Fourth, the public has always turned to clergy and religious persons in times of crisis, both clinical and developmental, to handle grief, marriage, family problems, the process of dying, moral and ethical education, and a great number of those existential and situational problems that face all living persons. In this decade, when an increasingly larger proportion of persons live beyond 55 years and face retirement, loss of meaningful work, and other problems in living, churches and synagogues are available and pastors and religiously trained persons are reachable to help elders resolve spiritual/psychological/social conflicts; herein lies the focus of psychotherapy.

The writer of Proverbs (23:7) said, "As a man thinketh in his heart, so is he." And General Douglas McArthur said in 1945,

> You don't get old by living a particular number of years; you get old when you desert your ideals. Years wrinkle your skin; renouncing your ideals wrinkles your soul. Worry, doubt, fear, are the enemies which slowly bring us down to the ground and turn us to dust before we die.

Paul Tournier, M.D., wrote in *Learn to Grow Old* (1972), "If one's old age is to be happy, there must be a change of attitude. Every false attitude, all disharmony in the person, will tend to get worse as the years go by and is pregnant with consequences for the future." Pastoral counseling deals with these nonmedical crises along with the aging progression in older persons and provides a vast resource for psychotherapy.

Recommended Readings

Arnold, A. *Guide yourself through old age.* Philadelphia: Fortress Press, 1976.

Clingan, D. F. *Aging persons in the community of faith.* St. Louis: Institute on Religion and Aging, Indiana Commission on the Aging and Aged, 1975.

Galton, L. *Don't give up on an aging parent.* New York: Crown Publishers, 1975.

Gray, R. M. and Moberg, D. O. *The church and the older person,* Rev. Ed. Grand Rapids, Mich.: William B. Eerdmans, 1977.

Herr, J. J. and Weakland, J. H. *Counseling elders and their families: practical techniques for applied gerontology.* New York: Springer, 1979.

Hiltner, S. *Toward a theology of aging.* New York: Human Sciences Press, 1975.

Howe, R. L. *How to stay younger while growing older; aging for all ages.* Waco, Texas: Word Books, 1974.

Maurus, J. *Growing old gracefully.* Canfield, Ohio: Alba Books, 1976.

Maves, P. B. and Cedarleaf, J. L. *Older people and the church.* Nashville: Abingdon Press, 1949.

Otte, E. *Welcome retirement.* St. Louis: Concordia Publishing House, 1974.

Poe, W. D. *The old person in your home.* New York: Scribner, 1969.

Stotsky, B. A. *The elderly patient.* New York: Grune and Stratton, 1968.

Tournier, P. *Learn to grow old.* New York: Harper and Row, 1972.

Part IV

Conclusions and Prospects

13

The Present and Future Role of Nontraditional Approaches

S. Stansfeld Sargent

This book has given a sampling of what we call "nontraditional therapy," positive programs now being conducted which circumvent the widespread senior resistance to psychotherapy and counseling. It is not a complete survey of the field; we had neither the time nor the money for this. But your editor thinks it is an impressive sampling. He is acquainted with nearly all the contributors personally and can vouch for the authenticity of the material presented. It provides evidence of a new, realistic, and encouraging trend to help older people solve their emotional problems and live more fulfilled lives.

Some Reasonable Questions

The reader, however, may have some doubts or questions as to the value or effectiveness of nontraditional therapy. Let us take up a few such queries and respond to them briefly but frankly. For example:

"*Granting that these approaches are probably helpful, should they be called* therapeutic? *Do they deal with the deep-seated problems of older people or just with the more superficial ones?*"

It is hard to generalize; the answer really depends on the motivation and defensiveness of the individuals themselves. A few people waste no time getting down to their major problem. Others seem to prefer to keep the involvement at a more superficial level; sometimes they get up and leave when things get too hot for them. With some, of course, the problem may *be* superficial. (One is reminded of the clinician who blurted out to his patient, "Your trouble is that you really *are* inferior!") Still others are uncertain at first but gradually feel comfortable enough to bring up the problem that bothers them most and to stay with it until they feel they have some kind of solution. Each of these is illustrated in cases cited by the contributors.

"How long do beneficial results last? How do you know people don't go right back to their old ways of feeling and behaving?"

One really doesn't know, as systematic follow-up is seldom done. Undoubtedly there are relapses, as with all counseling and psychotherapy. In a few of the cases reported, later chance meetings with the therapist occurred, and therapeutic benefits were found to have lasted over several months or even years. One encouraging feature is that, due to the good rapport established, persons who feel they were helped earlier often return to resume therapy when new problems arise.

"Do these newer approaches reach the older people who most need help?"

The answer to this, unfortunately, is mainly negative because the people most in need are often inaccessible and stoutly resistant to any contact or activity which might be therapeutic. On the other hand, nontraditional therapists are encouraged by sometimes being able to help people who have never asked for aid before, or whose contacts with more traditional therapy have been unsuccessful.

"Well then, do these nontraditional therapists reach enough older people to justify all the effort and expense involved?"

Nontraditional therapy is relatively new, experimental, variable, and difficult to assess in the sense of overall success. However, the answer is affirmative because many people are reached who have not been helped in other ways. Moreover, most of the programs are not very expensive to conduct, being carried out by volunteers, retired professionals, or by staff members as part of their regular assignment. A few programs have been fully or partially financed by grants.

"Might not these new kinds of approaches attract some distressed old people away from the professionals who are better qualified to help them?"

This is very doubtful in view of the typical senior resistance to "head doctors." Actually, the nontraditional therapist, after gaining rapport with older clients, is often the one who can best break through the resistance and bring about referral to a medical or psychological professional.

"Isn't there danger that volunteers or others with a minimum of training will think of themselves as psychotherapists and present themselves to the public in this way?"

There is always a chance that poorly trained people, or even worse, charlatans, will manage to gull the public. For this reason professional groups require licenses, set up standards, appoint review boards and the like. Training programs for peer counselors and other volunteers usually stress ethical standards and describe legal penalties for misrepresenting oneself to the public. Actually, the kind of persons who choose to get training in order to help our senior population are not the sort who try to make a "fast buck" by deceiving the public about their qualifications.

"But isn't this new therapy a kind of sugar-coated pill? And aren't we doing too much for the old folks anyway? Why don't we ask them to do more for themselves?"

As we have seen throughout the book, nontraditional therapy typically involves some degrees of indirection and disguise in order to circumvent the resistance shown by so many emotionally distressed older people. But it is not like a distant or impersonal agency which is doing something *to* the aging, or even *for* the aging. Like all good therapy and counseling, it works *with* aging individuals—with the aim of having the job taken over *by* these individuals themselves as soon as they feel up to it.

By Way of Summary

We who are doing nontraditional therapy certainly do not believe it is *the* solution to the emotional and human-relations problems of our senior population. It is one type of approach, which experiments, explores, and attempts to find new ways of reaching unhappy, frustrated, and distressed older people. The descriptions and cases we have presented here probably will not impress the scientifically minded who want quantitative results and statistical treatment. Perhaps funds will be available in the future for a research study of the effectiveness of nontraditional therapy with the aging, but to date such monies have not appeared.

In the meantime we believe our material provides models and fruitful suggestions for the growing number of persons who would like to furnish more therapeutic assistance to the aging. More specifically we submit that:

- it describes programs, activities, and resources of the sort already existing in many communities, to which distraught older persons or those interested in self-improvement can be referred for help (e.g., assertive training groups, widows' clubs, pastoral counselors, certain adult classes);
- it suggests new therapeutic approaches and modifications in ongoing programs and community facilities, such as rural discussion groups and workshops, behavioral techniques, day-care centers, nursing home orientation groups, peer counseling programs, self-actualizing workshops in the community;
- it indicates the kind of people—some professionals, some retirees, volunteers, paraprofessionals, some people in personal services—who are nonthreatening to seniors and who can be crucial in gaining their confidence and in motivating them to cope with their problems;
- it outlines the kind of training in counseling and therapeutic approaches which is essential for persons who wish to help older people but who need background, experience, and supervision;
- it suggests that, despite some initial apathy and suspicion, a significant segment of older people are reachable and are interested in learning and changing, in coping with their emotional difficulties, in warding off future troubles, and in living more satisfying lives;
- finally, it should encourage those who have been frustrated about not getting anywhere, therapeutically speaking, with older people. The contributors are not Pollyannas who think everything is "just lovely"; they are realists who have searched out ways to cope with many difficulties. Their efforts and achievements can give a boost to others who are working to help seniors solve their problems.

Now as to the Future

Certain ongoing trends seem especially relevant to the future prospects of nontraditional therapy.

First is the increasing longevity of our population, which is so well known by now it is hardly necessary to present actuarial figures. It is clear that we can expect a continuously growing number of older people and that they will live longer. More and more of them will be living 15, 20, even 25 and more years *after they retire,* which represents one-quarter to one-third of their whole life span. While this testifies to their improved health, we can assume that there will be many problems due to the higher cost of living and medical care in an era of continuing inflation and accelerating social change. Furthermore, one can assume a continuation if not an increase in emotional and human-relations problems. First Lady Rosalynn Carter was quoted in a news release of April 24, 1979, as saying that the President's Commission on Mental Health had found that though as many as 25 percent of the elderly might suffer from significant mental health problems, "very few actually receive treatment." Obviously all of our resources will be needed to meet the challenge of our expanding senior population.

It may be that senior resistance to psychotherapy is decreasing, which would mean more use of professional therapeutic services in the future. But the change is bound to be very gradual. The next generation of elders (people who are now middle-aged) seem more amenable to therapy and counseling than the present one, but they too are somewhat defensive and hardly enthusiastic about mental health services. Furthermore, when they reach retirement age they may begin to show some of the objections found in the current elders —e.g., lack of motivation for change, worry over cost of treatment, mobility and transportation problems, etc. On the other hand, there is some evidence that mental health professionals are becoming more interested in working with the aging, which makes the prospects somewhat more optimistic.

A parallel trend, probably arising from the growing participation by older people in educational, cultural, and community activities, is a burgeoning interest in preventive mental health services and activities, and more broadly in personal improvement and self-actualization.

All these suggest a continuing role for nontraditional types of therapy and counseling, though not necessarily in the form in which they exist today. In fact, we can be fairly sure they will be different, though it would be hard to predict their nature. The chances are good that many future programs will receive foundation support or government grants.

Perhaps we can do better at predicting who will provide the services, judging by present trends.

First, professionals in other than mental health fields will get further training and will provide more therapeutic services—e.g. nurses, social workers, teachers, physical and occupational therapists, and many others.

Retired persons with varying backgrounds—business, professional, artistic, secretarial, recreational—are already working as volunteers with the aging. Some of these are having training and are steering their activities in a therapeutic direction. The peer counselors are a particularly good example of this, but not the only one. Younger volunteers and paraprofessionals also are trying out ideas of their own, taking courses and attending institutes at gerontological centers.

Fortunately there seems to be a reciprocal growth of interest on the part of gerontologists. In the past their approach to "mental health of the aging" centered on organic and psychotic cases, many of them "senile" and mostly institutionalized. In recent years the literature has been marked by more attention to counseling and psychotherapy for noninstitutionalized older persons, though often without sufficient recognition of the problem of their resistance to treatment. The peer counseling program represents a real breakthrough here, since it centers on a distressed older person's acceptance of a peer—an elder "just like me" and a nonprofessional—who is interested, who listens, and who stands by in thick or thin.

Gerontological centers are growing rapidly and increasing their contacts with community agencies which deal with the aging. Volunteers and staff members from the agencies are taking courses and attending institutes; they are particularly interested in applied courses, of which those relating to counseling and therapy are quite popular. This trend can be seen in the listings of the gerontology centers at the University of Southern California, University of Michigan, Washington University, Duke University, and many other institutions, though their main emphasis is upon research, administration, and medical problems.

The Challenge of Nontraditional Therapy: A Final Word

In every community there are unhappy, distressed, unfulfilled older people who are not very accessible or cooperative or motivated for improvement. Up to now little effort has been made to reach them, but the nontraditional counselors and therapists have demonstrated that some of these people can be helped if one can only get through to them. These innovative workers have devised interesting and unusual programs and activities in order to break through the existing barriers of fear and resistance. They have worked hard with their unconventional approaches—which sometimes work and sometimes don't!

These pioneering people are an important leavening in a lumpy and hitherto barren area. Their successes and their failures, their efforts and their achievements, can stimulate us to take a fresh look at our own communities and their needs, borrowing and trying out some of the new techniques or programs which seem potentially useful. Or, even better, perhaps we can revise and improve them or work out something completely new, sharing our accomplishments later with our co-workers in other communities.

References

Aldrich, C. and Mendkoff, B. Relocation of the aged and disabled, a mortality study. *Journal of the American Geriatrics Society,* 1963, *11*, 185–194.

Alpaugh, P. and Haney, M. *Counseling the older adult—a training manual.* Los Angeles: Andrus Center, University of Southern California, 1978.

Atchley, R. C. *The social forces in later life.* Belmont, CA: Wadsworth, 1972.

Ayllon, T. and Houghton, E. Control of the behavior of schizophrenic patients by food. *Journal of the Experimental Analysis of Behavior,* 1962 *5,* 343–352.

Azrin, N. H. and Lindsley, O. R. The reinforcement of cooperation between children. *Journal of Abnormal and Social Psychology,* 1956, *52,* 100–102.

Beauvoir, S. de *The coming of age.* New York: Putnam, 1972.

Berry, J. A silent majority often unserved. *Perspective on Aging,* 1978, *7*, 24, 32.

Blake, R. Counseling in gerontology. *Personnel and Guidance Journal,* 1975, *53*, 733–737.

Blau, D. and Berezin, M. A. Neuroses and character disorders, Chapter 9. In J. G. Howells (Ed.). *Modern perspectives in the psychiatry of old age.* New York: Brunner-Mazel, 1975.

Blau, Z. S. *Old age in a changing society.* New York: New Viewpoints, 1973.

Blenkner, M. Environmental change and the aging individual. *Gerontologist,* 1967, *7*, 101–105.

Bocknek, G. A developmental approach to counseling adults. *Counseling Psychologist,* 1976, *6*, 37–40.

Brink, T. L. *Geriatric psychotherapy.* New York: Human Sciences Press, 1979.

Brody, E. M. *A social work guide for long-term care facilities.* Rockville, MD: National Institute for Mental Health, 1974.

Buckley, M. Counseling the aging. In J. R. Barry and C. R. Wingrove (Eds.). *Let's learn about aging.* Cambridge, MA: Schenkman, 1977.

Bultena, G. L. Rural-urban differences in the familial interaction of the aged. *Rural Sociology,* 1969, *34*, 5–15.

Butler, R. N. An interview with "Aging's Best Advocate." *APA Monitor* (American Psychological Association), 1976, *7*, 14.

Butler, R. N. Myths and realities of clinical geriatrics. *Image and Commentary,* 1970, *12*, 26–29.

Butler, R. N. *Why survive? Being old in America.* New York: Harper and Row, 1975.

Butler, R. N. and Lewis, M. I. *Aging and mental health; positive psychosocial approaches*, 2nd ed. St. Louis: C. V. Mosby, 1977.

Carp, F. The realities of interdisciplinary approaches: can the disciplines work together to help the aged? *In* A. N. Schwartz and I. Mensh (Eds.). *Professional obligations and approaches to the aged.* Springfield, IL: Thomas, 1974.

Cautela, J. R. A classical conditioning approach to the development and modification of behavior in the aged. *Gerontologist,* 1969, *9*, 109–113.

Cautela, J. R. and Kastenbaum, R. Assessment procedures for behavior modification with the aged. *Proceedings of the 20th Annual Meeting of the Gerontological Society,* 1967, *38*.

Clingan, D. F. *Aging persons in the community of faith.* St. Louis: Indiana Commission on the Aging and Aged, 1975.

Cohen, E. S. Legal research issues on aging. *Gerontologist,* 1974, *14*, 263–267.

Cohen, G. D. Mental health services and the elderly: needs and options. *American Journal of Psychiatry,* 1976, *133*, 65–68.

Collins, A. H. and Pancoast, D. L. *National helping networks.* Washington, D.C.: National Association of Social Work, 1976.

Comfort, A. *A good age.* New York: Simon and Schuster, 1976.

Davis, E. K. *Oral history*. Unpublished manuscript, 1975.

Davison, G. C. Appraisal of behavior modification techniques with adults in institutional settings. *In* C. M. Franks (Ed.). *Behavior therapy.* New York: McGraw-Hill, 1969.

Deeken, A. *Growing old and how to cope with it.* New York: Paulist Press, 1972.

Dychtwald, K. The Sage Project—a new image of age. *Journal of Humanistic Psychology,* 1978, *18*, 69–74.

Dye, C. Psychologist's role in the provision of mental health care for the elderly. *Professional Psychology,* 1978, *9*, 38–49.

Eisdorfer, C. and Lawton, M. P. (Eds.). *The psychology of adult development and aging.* Washington, D.C.: American Psychological Association, 1973.

Ellis, A. *Reason and emotion in psychotherapy.* New York: Lyle Stuart, 1962.

Erikson, E. H. *Childhood and society,* 2nd ed. New York: Norton, 1963.

Faulkner, A. O., Heisel, M. A., and Simms, P. Life strengths and life stresses: explorations in the measurement of the mental health of the black aged. *American Journal of Orthopsychiatry,* 1975, *45*, 102–110.

Ferster, C. B. and DeMyer, M. K. A method for the experimental analysis of the behavior of autistic children. *American Journal of Orthopsychiatry,* 1962, *32*, 89–98.

Frankl, V. *The doctor and the soul, an introduction to logotherapy.* New York: Knopf, 1955.

Gershon, M. and Biller, H. B. *The other helpers: paraprofessionals and nonprofessionals in mental health.* New York: Lexington Books, 1977.

Goldfried, M. R. and Davison, G. C. *Clinical behavior therapy.* New York: Holt, Reinhart and Winston, 1976.

Gray, R. M. and Moberg, D. O. *The church and the older person* (rev. ed.). Grand Rapids, MI: W. B. Eerdmans, 1977.

Gross, R., Gross, B., and Seidman, S. (Eds.). *The new old: struggling for decent aging.* New York: Anchor Books, 1978.

Guthrie, E. R. *The psychology of learning.* (rev. ed.). New York: Harper and Row, 1952.

Harlow, H. E. The formation of learning sets. *Psychological Review,* 1949, *56*, 51–65.

Harrison, L. and Entine, A. Existing programs and emerging strategies. *Counseling Psychologist,* 1976, *6,* #1.

Harrison, W. R. Old age homes: gilded cages for domesticated canaries. *Geriatric Focus,* 1970, *9* (3), 1–4.

Hiltner, S. *Toward a theology of aging.* New York: Human Sciences Press, 1975.

Hoyer, W. J., Mishara, B. L., and Riebel, R. G. Problem behaviors as operants: applications with elderly individuals. *Gerontologist,* 1975, *15*, 452–456.

Hurvitz, N. Peer self-help psychotherapy groups and their implications for psychotherapy. *Psychotherapy: Theory and Research,* 1970, *7*, 4–49.

Jasnau, K. F. Individualized versus mass transfer of non-psychotic geriatric patients from mental hospitals to nursing homes, with special reference to death rate. *Journal of the American Geriatrics Society,* 1967, *15*, 280–284.

Kahn, R. L. Perspectives in the evaluation of psychological mental health problems for the aged. *In* W. D. Gentry (Ed.). *Geropsychology: a model of training and clinical service.* Cambridge, MA: Ballinger, 1977.

Kahn, R. L. The mental health system and the future aged. *Gerontologist,* 1975, *15*, 24–31.

Kahn, R. L. and Zarit, S. H. Evaluation of mental health programs for the aged. *In* P. O. Davidson, F. W. Clark, and L. A. Hammerlynek (Eds.). *Evaluation of behavioral programs.* Champaign: Research Press, 1974.

Kalish, R. A. *Late adulthood: perspectives on human development.* Monterey, CA: Brooks/Cole, 1975.

Kassabaum, G. E. Shaping environment to enhance life and service. Paper presented at Lutheran Conference on Services to the Aging, St. Louis, MO, 1969.

Kastenbaum, R. The reluctant therapist. *In* R. Kastenbaum (Ed.). *New thoughts on old age.* New York: Springer, 1964.

King, G. F., Armitage, S. G., and Tilton, J. R. A therapeutic approach to schizophrenics of extreme pathology. *Journal of Abnormal and Social Psychology,* 1960, *61*, 276–286.

Kobrynski, B. The mentally impaired elderly—whose responsibility? *Gerontologist,* 1975, *15*, 407.

Lawton, M. P. The impact of environment on aging and behavior. *In* J. E. Birren and K. W. Schaie (Eds.). *Handbook of the psychology of aging.* New York: Litton, 1977, pp. 276–301.

Lawton, M. P. and Gottesman, L. E. Psychological services to the elderly. *American Psychologist,* 1974, *29*, 689–693.

Libb, J. W. and Clements, B. Token reinforcement in an exercise program for hospitalized geriatric patients. *Perceptual and Motor Skills,* 1969, *2* (3) 957–958.

Lieberman, M. Institutionalization of the aged: effects on behavior. *Journal of Gerontology,* 1969, *24*, 330–340.

Lieberman, M. Relationship of mortality rates to entrance to a home for the aged. *Geriatrics,* 1961, *16*, 515–519.

Lieberman, M. and Lakin, M. On becoming an institutionalized aged person. *In* R. Williams, C. Tibbitts, and W. Donahue (Eds.). *Processes of aging.* Englewood Cliffs, NJ: Prentice-Hall, 1963.

Lieberman, M., Prock, V. N., and Tobin, S. S. Psychological effects of institutionalization. *Journal of Gerontology,* 1968, *23,* 343–353.

Linden, M. Group psychotherapy with institutionalized senile women: study in gerontologic human relations. *International Journal of Group Psychotherapy,* 1953, *3*, 150–170.

Lindsley, O. R. Geriatric behavioral prosthetics. *In* R. Kastenbaum (Ed.). *New thoughts on old age.* New York: Springer, 1964.

Lipsett, D. R. A medical-psychological approach to dependence in the aged. *In* R. A. Kalish (Ed.). *The dependencies of old people.* Ann Arbor: Institute of Gerontology, University of Michigan-Wayne State University, 1969.

Markus, E., Blenkner, M., and Downs, T. Some factors and their association with post-relocation mortality among institutionalized aged persons. *Journal of Gerontology,* 1972, *27*, 376–382.

Maslow, A. H. *Motivation and personality.* New York: Harper and Row, 1954.

Maslow, A. H. *Toward a psychology of being,* 2nd ed. Princeton, NJ: Van Nostrand, 1968.

Maurus, J. *Growing old gracefully.* Canfield, OH: Alba Books, 1976.

McClellan, R. W. *Claiming a frontier; ministry and older people.* Berkeley: University of California Press, 1977.

McKean, M. Seniors: they talked of emotions, sexuality, feelings, Ventura, CA: Star-Free Press, Sec. B-1, Oct. 23, 1977.

Mishler, K. Of people and pigeons. *S.K.&F. Psychiatric Reporter,* 1964, #15.

Moberg, D. O. Needs felt by the clergy for ministries to the aging. *Gerontologist,* 1975, *15*, 170–175.

Moberg, D. O. The church-synagogue hearing the challenge in making the knowledge explosion work for the elderly. 19th Annual Meeting, Western Gerontological Society, 1973.

Moen, E. The reluctance of the elderly to accept help. *Social Problems,* 1978, *25*, 293–303.

Moriarty, D. M. (Ed.). *The loss of loved ones; the effects of a death in the family on personality development.* Springfield, IL: Thomas, 1967.

Morris, J. N. Changes in morale experienced by elderly institutional applicants along the institutional path. *Gerontologist,* 1975, *15*, 345–349.

Noll, P. F. An alphabet soup of agencies fails. *Perspectives on Aging,* 1978, *7*: 19–23.

Oden, T. A populists's view of psychotherapeutic deprofessionalization. *Journal of Humanistic Psychology,* 1974, *14*, 2, 3–18.

Paul, G. L. Chronic mental patient: current status—future directions. *Psychological Bulletin,* 1969, *71*, 81–94.

Philblad, C. T. and Rosencranz, H. A. *Social adjustment of older people in the small town.* Columbia, MO: University of Missouri Press, 1969.

Poe, W. D. *The old person in your home.* New York: Scribner, 1967.

Pressey, S. L. Age counseling: crises, services, potentials. *Journal of Counseling Psychology,* 1973, *20,* 356–360.

Pressey, S. L. and Pressey, S. D. Major neglected need opportunity: old age counseling. *Journal of Counseling Psychology,* 1972, *19*, 362–366.

Randall, O. A. Aging in American today—new aspects in aging. *Gerontologist,* 1977, *17*, 6–11.

Reiff, R. and Riessman, F. The indigenous nonprofessional: a strategy of change in community action and community health programs. *Community Mental Health Journal,* 1965, Monograph #1.

Rioch, M. J. Changing concepts in the training of therapists. *Journal of Consulting Psychology,* 1966, *30*, 290–292.

Rioch, M., Elkes, C., Flint, A. A., Usdansky, S., Newman, R. G., and Silber, E. National Institute of Mental Health pilot study in training mental health counselors. *American Journal of Orthopsychiatry,* 1963, *33* (4), 678–689.

Rogers, C. R. The necessary and sufficient conditions of therapeutic personality change. *Journal of Consulting Psychology,* 1957, *21*, 95–103.

Samuelson, R. Is the graying of the federal budget inevitable? *Los Angeles Times,* March 12, 1978.

Sarton, M. *Plant dreaming deep.* New York: Norton, 1968.

Schaie, K. W. and Griffin, K. Adult development and ageing. *Annual Review of Psychology,* 1975, *26*, 65–96.

Schlossberg, N. The case for counseling adults. *Counseling Psychologist,* 1976, *6*, 33–36.

Schwartz, A. N. *Survival handbook for children of aging parents.* Chicago: Follett, 1977.

Shanas, E. and Maddox, G. L. Aging and health resources—study of physical and mental health status of the elderly. *In* R. H. Binstock and E. Shanas (Eds.). *Handbook of aging and the social sciences.* New York: Van Nostrand, 1976.

Simon, S. B., Howe, L. W., and Kirschenbaum, H. *Values clarification.* New York: Hart Publishing Co., 1972.

Skinner, B. F. *Beyond freedom and dignity.* New York: Knopf, 1971.

Skinner, B. F. *Science and human behavior.* New York: Macmillan, 1953.

Smith, M. J. *When I say No, I feel guilty.* New York: Bantam, 1975.

Sobey, F. *The non-professional revolution in mental health.* New York: Columbia University Press, 1970.

Stotsky, B. A. *The elderly patient.* New York: Grune and Stratton, 1968.

Stuart, R. B. *Behavioral self-management.* New York: Brunner/Mazel, 1977.

Swenson, E. W. The effect of instruction and reinforcement on the behavior of geriatric psychiatric patients. (Doctoral dissertation, University of Utah, 1965). *Dissertation Abstracts,* 1966, *26*(8).

Swenson, E. W. The effect of instruction and reinforcement on the behavior of geriatric psychiatric patients. *In* R. D. Rubin, H. Fensterheim, A. A. Lazarus, and C. M. Franks (Eds.). *Advances in behavior therapy.* New York: Academic Press, 1971.

Swenson, E. W. and Rosenstein, J. C. More services to more people. *Viewpoints,* 1978, *3*, 26–28.

Taves, I. *Women alone.* New York: Funk and Wagnalls, 1968.

Tharp, G. R. and Wetzel, R. J. *Behavioral modification in the natural environment.* New York: Academic Press, 1969.

Tilton, J. R. The use of instrumental motor and verbal learning techniques in the treatment of chronic schizophrenics. Unpublished doctoral dissertation, Michigan State University, 1956.

Toseland, R. and Sykes, J. Senior citizens center participation and other correlates of life satisfaction. *Gerontologist,* 1977, *17*, 235–241.

Tournier, P. *Learn to grow old.* New York: Harper and Row, 1972.

Troll, L. and Nowak, C. How old are your?—The question of age bias in the counseling of adults. *Counseling Psychologist,* 1976, *6*, 41–44.

Truax, C. and Carkhuff, R. *Toward effective counseling and psychotherapy: training and practice.* Chicago: Aldine, 1967.

Twente, E. E. *Never too old.* San Francisco: Jossey-Bass, 1970.

Tyler, L. *The work of the counselor,* 3rd ed. New York: Appleton-Century-Crofts, 1969.

Varah, C. (Ed.). *The Samaritans.* New York: Macmillan, 1965.

Wahler, H. J., Johnson, R., and Uhrich, K. *The community mental health expediter project.* Olympia: Department of Social and Health Services, State of Washington, 1972.

Waters, E. and White, B. Helping each other. In L. E. Troll, J. Israel, and K. Israel, (Eds.). *Looking ahead; a woman's guide to the problems and joys of growing older.* Englewood Cliffs, N.J.: Prentice-Hall, 1977.

Wolff, K. Treatment of the geriatric patient in a mental hospital. *Journal of the American Geriatric Society,* 1956, *4*, 472–476.

Young, R. K. and Meiburg, A. L. *Spiritual therapy—how the physician, psychiatrist and minister collaborate in healing.* New York: Harper and Row, 1960.

Index